T0203031

Research Methods for
Student Radiographers

Medical Imaging in Practice

Series Editor: Christopher Hayre, Senior Lecturer in Diagnostic Radiography, Charles Sturt University, Australia.

Research Methods for Student Radiographers: A Survival Guide
Christopher M. Hayre and Xiaoming Zheng

For more information about this series, please visit:
https://www.crcpress.com/Medical-Imaging-in-Practice/book-series/MIIP

Research Methods for Student Radiographers

A Survival Guide

Christopher M. Hayre and Xiaoming Zheng

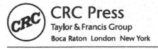

CRC Press
Taylor & Francis Group
Boca Raton London New York

CRC Press is an imprint of the
Taylor & Francis Group, an **informa** business

First edition published 2022
by CRC Press
2 Park Square, Milton Park, Abingdon, Oxon OX14 4RN

and by CRC Press
6000 Broken Sound Parkway NW, Suite 300, Boca Raton, FL 33487-2742

© 2022 Christopher M. Hayre, Xiaoming Zheng

CRC Press is an imprint of Informa UK Limited

British Library Cataloguing-in-Publication Data
A catalogue record for this book is available from the British Library

Library of Congress Cataloging-in-Publication Data
Names: Hayre, Christopher M., author. | Zheng, Xiaoming, author.
Title: Research methods for student radiographers: a survival
guide / Christopher M. Hayre, Xiaoming Zheng.
Description: First edition. | Boca Raton : CRC Press, 2022. |
Series: Medical imagining in practice | Includes bibliographical references and index. |
Summary: "This book aims to provide a holistic picture of the application of research in
radiography focusing on the multi-variant methodological approaches and practices.
It will provide readers with an insight into both contemporary and innovative methods within
radiography, backed up with existing evidence-based research"– Provided by publisher.
Identifiers: LCCN 2021019182 (print) | LCCN 2021019183 (ebook) |
ISBN 9780367558710 (hardback) | ISBN 9780367559335 (paperback) |
ISBN 9780367559311 (ebook)
Subjects: LCSH: Radiography, Medical–Methodology.
Classification: LCC RC78 .H39 2022 (print) |
LCC RC78 (ebook) | DDC 616.07/572–dc23
LC record available at https://lccn.loc.gov/2021019182
LC ebook record available at https://lccn.loc.gov/2021019183

ISBN: 978-0-367-55871-0 (hbk)
ISBN: 978-0-367-55933-5 (pbk)
ISBN: 978-0-367-55931-1 (ebk)

DOI: 10.1201/9780367559311

Typeset in Times
by Newgen Publishing UK

Dr. Christopher Hayre would like to dedicate this book to Charlotte, Ayva, Evelynn and Ellena. He would also like to dedicate this book to family members back home and to Professor Dave Muller for making it all possible.

Dr. Xiaoming Zheng would like to dedicate this book to Xiaodan, Rachel and Charlotte. He would also like to dedicate this book to his extended family overseas.

Contents

Acknowledgments...xi
Author Biographies..xiii
Preface...xv

Chapter 1 Introducing Research Methods for Student Radiographers 1

    1.1   Introduction..1
    1.2   What Is Research and What Does It Offer?...............................2
    1.3   What Are Research Paradigms?..5
            1.3.1   Quantitative Research..7
            1.3.2   Qualitative Research..7
    1.4   Three p's to Engaging in the Research Process 8
    1.5   Contemporary Context for Radiography Research...................9
    1.6   Chapter Summary 11
    Key Terms..11
    Exercises and Study Questions..12

Chapter 2 Philosophical Foundations for Radiography Research 15

    2.1   Introduction..15
    2.2   What Is Research Philosophy?..16
    2.3   Philosophy of Experimental Researchers 18
    2.4   Philosophy of Naturalistic Researchers 21
    2.5   Philosophy for Mixed Method Researchers............................26
    2.6   Philosophy for Radiographic Researchers? 27
    2.7   Chapter Summary 28
    Key Terms..28
    Exercises and Study Questions..30

Chapter 3 Research Essentials in Diagnostic Radiography 33

    3.1   Introduction..33
    3.2   Conceptualizing and Contextualizing the Research
            Problem..33
    3.3   Evaluate Existing Literature...36
    3.4   The 'Problem' or 'Opportunity' and Research Questions 39
    3.5   Analysing, Mapping and Drawing Conclusions 39
    3.6   Chapter Summary 42
    Key Terms..43
    Exercises and Study Questions..43

Chapter 4 Ethical Considerations in Radiography Research 45

    4.1   Introduction 45
    4.2   Role of Research Ethics and Historical Context 45
    4.3   Principles Protecting Human Participants 47
          4.3.1   Disclosure 48
          4.3.2   Confidentiality 49
          4.3.3   Participation 50
          4.3.4   Consent 53
    4.4   Post Study Approval and Monitoring 55
    4.5   Does the Ethical Process Stop? 56
    4.6   Chapter Summary 58
    Key Terms 59
    Exercises and Study Questions 60

Chapter 5 Quantitative Approaches for Radiography 63

    5.1   Introduction 63
    5.2   Rationale for Quantitative Approaches 63
    5.3   X-ray Experimental Designs 65
    5.4   Non-experimental Designs 67
    5.5   Epidemiology 70
    5.6   Clinical Trial Methodology 72
    5.7   Chapter Summary 74
    Key Terms 75
    Exercises and Study Questions 76

Chapter 6 Data Collection in Quantitative Research 79

    6.1   Introduction 79
    6.2   Measurement Process 79
    6.3   Experimental Data Collection Strategies 82
    6.4   Non-experimental Data Collection Strategies 85
    6.5   Ensuring Methodological Reliability and Validity 88
    6.6   Chapter Summary 89
    Key Terms 90
    Exercises and Study Questions 90

Chapter 7 Statistical Analysis in Quantitative Research 93

    7.1   Introduction 93
    7.2   Why Do We Need Statistics? 93
    7.3   Descriptive Statistics 94
    7.4   Inferential Statistics 98
    7.5   Chapter Summary 104
    Key Terms 105
    Exercises and Study Questions 105

Chapter 8   Qualitative Approaches for Radiography 109

      8.1   Introduction 109
      8.2   The Value of Qualitative Approaches 110
      8.3   Ethnography 112
      8.4   Phenomenology 115
      8.5   Grounded Theory 117
      8.6   Action Research 119
      8.7   Chapter Summary 122
      Key Terms 122
      Exercises and Study Questions 123

Chapter 9   Data Collection in Qualitative Research 127

      9.1   Introduction 127
      9.2   Establishing Ethical and Moral Boundaries 127
      9.3   Data Collection Methods 129
            9.3.1   Observations 129
            9.3.2   Interviews 130
            9.3.3   Focus Groups 133
      9.4   Where and When Is it Ok to Collect Data? 135
      9.5   Researcher Positionality and Reflexivity 136
      9.6   Chapter Summary 139
      Key Terms 140
      Exercises and Study Questions 141

Chapter 10   Data Analysis and Trustworthiness in Qualitative Research 145

      10.1   Introduction 145
      10.2   Qualitative Data Analysis 146
            10.2.1   Computer-Aided Versus Non-Computer-
                       Aided Analysis 146
            10.2.2   Note-Taking: A Data Collection and
                       Analytical Process 148
            10.2.3   'Getting Ready': Things to Consider 148
            10.2.4   The Beginnings of Data Analysis 149
            10.2.5   Thematic Analysis 151
             10.2.6   Constant Comparative Method 153
            10.2.7   Analysis in Phenomenological Research 155
      10.3   Trustworthiness of Data 156
            10.3.1   Credibility 157
            10.3.2   Transferability 159
            10.3.3   Dependability 160
            10.3.4   Confirmability 162
            10.3.5   Authenticity 163

10.4   Chapter Summary 164
Key Terms.. 165
Exercises and Study Questions... 166

Chapter 11 What Next?.. 171

11.1   Introduction.. 171
11.2   Leaving the Field 171
11.3   Impact of Research 173
11.4   Reflexive Practitioner... 176
11.5   Monitoring 178
11.6   Chapter Summary 179
Key Terms.. 179
Exercises and Study Questions... 181

Chapter 12 Book Summary.. 183

Index 185

Acknowledgments

The authors of this book would like to begin by acknowledging our undergraduate and postgraduate students. Our combined experiences of teaching and learning to diagnostic radiography students at an undergraduate and postgraduate level have led to the development of this book. The authors would also like to thank one another for what has been an enjoyable and celebratory project. As an authored book, we have learnt from one another, as well as ourselves in producing this text. The collegial view as both a diagnostic radiographer [CH] and medical physicist [XZ], we feel it has not only enhanced the scholarly nature of this work, but also exemplifies our appreciation and motivation for pursing our own scholarly goals. Lastly, a special thank you to Mark Filmer for his assistance in editing some of the contents of this book and also Heba Gumaa for the illutrations.

Author Biographies

Dr. Christopher M. Hayre is currently a Senior Lecturer in Diagnostic Radiography at Charles Sturt University in New South Wales, Australia. He has published both qualitative and quantitative refereed papers in the field of Diagnostic Radiography and has brought together a number of edited books in the field of health research, everyday technology and ethnography. He founded the *Journal of Social Science & Allied Health Professions* in 2016 and remains Editor-in-Chief. He is currently working on books pertinent to the radiographic profession and has recently been made Editor of his own book series, Medical Imaging in Practice by Taylor & Francis.

Dr. Xiaoming Zheng has been teaching medical radiation science courses at Charles Sturt University since 1998. He was a medical physicist at the Prince of Wales Hospital Sydney prior to his appointment at CSU. He earned a PhD in physics from the University of Newcastle and subsequently worked as a postdoctoral fellow in applied mathematics at the University of Wollongong and lecturer A in theoretical chemistry at the University of Sydney. Dr. Zheng grew up in China and was educated at Zhejiang University China where he earned his Bachelor and Master degrees and held an assistant lecturer position. He also spent seven months at the University of Massachusetts Medical School USA on a special study leave.

Preface

This book, just like any research project, takes the researcher on a journey. This journey is based on two experienced researchers that, although stem from two separate disciplines, collectively share a common goal – the undertaking and dissemination of radiography research. As this book has progressed, coincided with close engagement with one another, it is apparent that collaboration is not only key, but it is through those collaborative efforts with peers that we enhance our dialogue, engagement and thinking – a central component of this book. Then, we decided to develop a 'research guide' because whilst having taught undergraduate, postgraduate and supervised PhD students, we felt this book could 'signpost' students by reflecting on our experiences to date. Further, our transnational involvement in research projects over the years brings an international lens to this book and thus anticipates the narrative to resonate with others worldwide.

This text is primarily focused on students studying research methods at an undergraduate level, but may also resonate with students studying at either masters or doctoral level. Whilst this remains our primary audience, there will be other health disciplines that may find chapters insightful. For instance, chapter 2 discusses philosophical considerations that can be applied across the health spectrum and in a cross-discipline manner. Further, prospective methodological and researcher considerations may also help refocus or rethink previous ideas or strategies, depending on the researcher's intention. As methodological frameworks, tools, coupled with quantitative and qualitative analysis are discussed, we will integrate our own research throughout. This is important because whilst the book primarily speaks to a radiography community, it may also spark interest from other groups. For practitioners seeking to either assert some empirical rationale to their everyday observations or consider engaging in research in the clinical environment, they may also find this text helpful in guiding and identifying research problems and importantly, executing them clinically.

As indicated above, this book does not seek to replace nor become a primary book of choice. Our view is that this book simply offers a supplementary, and perhaps at times controversial view of radiographic research. It is important to recognize that whilst some of our narrative and ideas may be viewed as commonplace, this does not always lead to acceptance. As researchers, practitioners and educators, we not only wish to examine questions and seek out answers, but also seek to challenge the status quo, providing novel ways of 'thinking and doing' in order to prevent confinement and dogmatic beliefs. It is anticipated that this book not only offers supplementary views on our current understanding and practices towards radiography research, but also seeks, on occasion, to dismantle 'ways of thinking and doing' from a reflexive process that seeks to inform future methodological and empirical research in radiography.

Dr. Christopher M. Hayre

Dr. Xiaoming Zheng

1 Introducing Research Methods for Student Radiographers

Christopher M. Hayre

1.1 INTRODUCTION

This introductory chapter sets the scene for first-time researchers who have either enrolled or are undertaking some form of empirical research. In part, this chapter introduces the reader to some basic questions, such as 'what is research?' and 'what are research paradigms?' These are important in terms of clarifying any presumptions previously held, but also links to future questions around research in diagnostic radiography. For undergraduate radiography students entering the research context for the first time, they are often exposed to unique terms and phrases, which remain unfamiliar. As this chapter progresses, however, it will introduce these terms to situate both quantitative and qualitative research. It will also provide some rationale and grounding in terms of recognizing that research approaches are often polarized. This leads to my own motivation in developing this book in an attempt to expose uncertainties for students, which can later be challenged and/or applied in the academic space. This chapter not only asserts the value of research amongst radiography students and any prospective practitioners, it also outlines the value of research within our profession, now, and in future years. Whilst this book is principally a text for the undergraduate audience, it will also resonate with practitioners, postgraduate students and perhaps academic staff entering higher education employment for the first time. From experience, we may often work with peers who have extensive or little research experience; practitioners leaving clinical work and entering higher education for either study or employment are commonplace. This chapter speaks to those individuals. Interestingly, this book may be used by practicing radiographers who are thinking of starting a research project whilst in their clinical role. The latter engagement is potentially more exciting whereby the practice of research amongst practicing radiographers is an 'everyday role'.

This chapter (and forthcoming chapters) is based on teaching, learning and research experiences. Having taught and researched in several parts of the world, this book offers a transnational 'feel' towards the practice and application of research in radiography. Central in this process is reflexivity, which intertwines the practice of research with self-development, which is not static, but develops and re-develops as time progresses. This chapter will introduce key terms affiliated with each research

DOI: 10.1201/9780367559311-1

methodology in order for students to become familiar with them. It will also set the stage for subsequent chapters within this book and signpost accordingly, whilst also making reference to other key texts throughout. There is also a potential caveat. As the book progresses, subsequent chapters and the overall narrative will also evolve, as does any research project. This is important to highlight now as it may be considered a juxtaposition, which we reject. For instance, there are instances in this book that are written in a context that is generally accepted, i.e., the norm or convention. This is important for new researchers in order to understand the 'general feel' of what it means to talk and discuss about research processes. The use of inverted commas not only emphasizes but also illustrates that logic can change or even be misplaced. For instance, whilst discussion around certain methodologies is written to a level of acceptable understandings at levels 4 and 5 for higher education purposes, it is also important to challenge dogmatic views and approaches in our contemporary space. This does not mean it is correct, nor should it be dismissed, but through evidence base knowledge and peer review, this book, at times, professes alternate viewpoints that may allow the reader to express or challenge their own research agenda(s) and/or previous conventions as they 'journey' throughout their own research. After all, radiography is positioned within the social sciences and natural sciences and to reject the use of either social science or natural science would arguably disregard the distinct and unique scope of radiography research being conducted. We even propose radiography as a 'united science' whereby radiography and prospective researchers not only appreciate the value of each paradigmatic tradition, but observe the utility and egalitarian motives in order to advance our profession forward.

1.2   WHAT IS RESEARCH AND WHAT DOES IT OFFER?

In order to begin to answer the question 'what research is?' it is important to introduce the term 'originality'. As a radiography student, reading this book, you would have been exposed to a wealth of existing literature within your tertiary education setting. This knowledge informs your education and is today published in a number of formats: authored textbooks (like this one), edited book volumes, journal articles and conference proceedings. This 'evidence' is encapsulated within what we term, an evidence base, paradigm and/or body of knowledge. They are interchangeable, yet the term paradigm is generally interpreted as a standard perspective, or a set of ideas concerning a discipline existing at a particular point in time (Kuhn, 1962). This current knowledge base manifests itself in a number of ways. For instance, it may encompass understandings, such as how X-ray tubes operate, or the known radiobiological interactions/effects within tissues and/or perhaps how digital radiographs are produced, and then optimized via amorphous selenium (a-Se) detectors (Hayre and Cox, 2020). These concepts exist within our radiographic body of knowledge or radiographic paradigm, along with many other schools of thought and concepts. This notion of 'knowing what we know' offers an important lens in order to gain an understanding of what research means for us as a profession as we seek to uncover what we do not know.

Research is typically defined as the creation of new knowledge or use of existing knowledge, but applied in a new and creative way, which can instil new ways of thinking whilst applying alternate methodologies (O'Reilly, 2011). For instance, this may involve critically examining previously published literature and challenging new ideas or suggestions for future research. In addition, the concept of undertaking empirical research is underscored by adding information, adding something new, which has either, say, been acquired by participant observation or X-ray experimentation. Another way of understanding research is understanding our need for empiricism. Empiricism in the general sense sits within qualitative and quantitative paradigms, but is principally aligned with epistemological theory and regarded as the source of knowledge (Adams, 1975). This is discussed in more detail in chapter 2. As researchers, then, our intention is seeking out new empiricism, thus seeking new knowledge. For diagnostic radiography, this does not always mean setting up an X-ray experiment and recording photons in a controlled way. As we will come to appreciate, research enables us to develop our knowledge, our current schools of thinking, challenge customary beliefs, behaviours and attitudes, and perhaps going against conventional norms. These aspects of research, then, requires a number of tools (which we will recognize as research methods) in order to not only appreciate the varied nature of the world around us, but also the utilization of varied (and often opposing) strategies to help us advance our knowledge and provide innovative ways of performing research.

When we think of the word data in radiography, we want readers to not directly link this to numbers on a spreadsheet, which can later be used for statistical inference. Whilst important and identified in chapters 5–7, this book recognizes that data can involve words, sentences, pictures, and reflections – discussed more in chapters 8–10. Further, whilst the authors of this text have their own research goals and pursuits, we respect data emanating from appropriately applied research strategies, grounded by their respective paradigmatic traditions and associated philosophies, regardless of their qualitative or quantitative nature. Griffiths and Norman (2013, p.583) highlight that in the field of nursing, a 'paradigm war' has the possibility of hindering academic development. As paradigmatic disagreements exist in other fields, such as nursing, we may also hear and/or observed similar rhetoric in radiography whereby one paradigm is favoured amongst academics, or seen as superior, over another.

Whilst we accept these paradigmatic traditions as methodological, any engagement with the research process in terms of offering value should enable researchers to 'break out' of what has already been defined as the epistemological paradigm. This is important. By breaking out, its synonymous with the term originality and reinforces what research is and what it can offer. For those reading and embarking onto honours, masters or doctoral study, the volume and level of 'breaking out' [originality], coupled with epistemological relevance will naturally differ. The latter awards naturally demand greater contribution and originality to the profession and, above all, dissemination. Prior to seeking any new information for your own level of intended study, it is important to ask: what level of originality is expected and will it be enough? Ongoing discussions with your supervisory team and colleagues will remain central as there is now a general acceptance that researchers are expected to have published prior to embarking onto PhD programmes. This is certainly a paradigm shift when comparing and considering, say, a PhD to be an apprenticeship in research, which certainly remained the case for the first author upon entering his PhD studentship programme in the United Kingdom. Currently, there is perhaps greater expectation on prospective students to whom have already gained research experience in order to become successful PhD Candidates.

For the research process itself, there should be a chronological framework in terms of how we, the authors, feel the research process can be approached, in terms of conceptualizing, as well as performing research. For instance, forthcoming chapters examine philosophical underpinnings (chapter 2), usually a requirement of consideration during developmental phases. Next, the development of research questions, aims and objectives (chapter 3), which is followed up with identifying ethical considerations in chapter 4. The book, then, focuses on methodological considerations for quantitative approaches (chapters 5–7), supported with qualitative approaches (chapters 8–10). Chapter 11 considers aspects relevant to the researcher post data collection and analysis such as leaving the field, research impact and consideration of the reflexive practitioner. These discussions are not only outcomes as a result of reflexive processes during the development of this book, but also intend to demonstrate an outlook on self and how this could be transferable.

The delivery and style of this book could readily be applied for teaching and learning delivery, supplemented with other key texts. Yet, the design, on initial examination does not appreciate reflexivity. Like most books, it is important to demonstrate chapters chronologically, e.g., chapters 1–11 in this case; however, it is argued that researchers go beyond this linear model when conducting, analysing and publishing results. Instead, it is recognized that the research process requires moving 'back and forth' theoretically, analytically and practically, in some circumstances, regardless of the strategy employed. This perspective is explained in more detail in chapters 9 and 11, the former engaging in the process of reflexivity as a data collection tool, with the latter considering reflexivity for learners and practitioners. In short, it is not presupposed that reflexivity remains a process considered simply 'at the end' of any research process, quite the contrary. As this book evolved, we also encourage readers to recognize the fluid state of research, coincided with the importance of continuously engaging with the literature, meeting supervisors (individually and collectively), supported clinical experiences, upgrade meetings and/or simply conversations with peers. These remain central to the development of the research project, thesis and, most importantly, you as the researcher. It is acknowledged that any process or direction in which a student initially embarks upon is not linear and that alternate paths may be necessary and unavoidable. Instances, then, of backtracking or sidestepping may be necessary in order to ensure a successful project. For now, as we delve into the early stages of research it is recommended we continue with a linear approach, but also appreciate changes and deviances along the way.

Because this book is focused on assisting undergraduate researchers, as supervisors of undergraduate, postgraduate and PhD students, we understand the unknown and often challenging situations students find themselves in. Whilst the title of this book indicates some form of survival need to progress, it is important that students utilize the skills and knowledge of their PhD supervisors as they are often central in guiding and directing. So, when asked, 'what is research and what does it offer?' it is evident that the practice of undertaking research and publishing original data is clearly paramount, yet, as acknowledged, the research journey also embodies the student, the profession and career aspirations of individuals seeking to move into the research or academic world.

1.3 WHAT ARE RESEARCH PARADIGMS?

In order to set aside and discern differences between quantitative and qualitative research, it is important to think of the basics. Whilst there may be overlap, whereby quantitative methods can be used to collect qualitative data (and vice versa), for the purposes of understanding differing approaches let us highlight some basic components. For example, when we think of quantitative methods, we are typically focused on collating data in a numerical format. Qualitative research, on the other hand, is generally accepted as research that observes natural settings and collects actions, narratives or pictorial evidence of certain phenomenon (Saks and Allsop, 2010). In radiography, we use both and each offers value and insight within our literature. Thus, whilst we appreciate the overarching acceptance and use of such approaches, they hold different assumptions. For instance, in qualitative research, we typically do not seek breadth, but depth, on a particular topic or idea (Hammersley and Atkinson, 2007). Qualitative researchers are not particularly interested in variables, which are necessary for performing X-ray experiments, for instance. Qualitative researchers are principally interested in the varied, unique and ungeneralizable events occurring in the everyday environment. This is why qualitative researchers may align themselves to the social sciences, a field of research that seeks to uncover human behaviour, attitudes and opinions of individuals within a particular context and at a particular moment in time.

When speaking to students for the first time about what it means to do research, it often leads to the same analogy – a swimming pool. By linking a swimming pool it can represent our body of knowledge. Let's be imaginative for a moment. Let us consider our current understandings (evidence) have been printed and thrown into a swimming pool. Then, in order to ensure we uncover this evidence, we then immerse ourselves in the pool and start to understand the literature. Let's now imagine that after some time in the pool you have gathered enough evidence and become intellectually poised to understand the existing knowledge pertinent to your project or area of expertise. At this stage, you may think about exiting the pool. Upon looking back at the pool your perspective will have naturally altered thus allowing you to discern perhaps some original thought from an initial idea. The pool analogy helps us depict the paradigm, as illustrated in Figure 1.1 – the bounds of our current knowledge, but also how, as researchers, our perspectives change when we later emerged. The same can be associated with research paradigms whereby our alternate schools of thought seek to uncover novel findings.

Below are three reflective points refining what we have discussed thus far, coincided with affirming what research is and the key attributes required if originality is to be sought:

1   *Research should be adding something new to the discipline, thus expanding the paradigm and building our evidence base knowledge – i.e., the area not found in the swimming pool.*

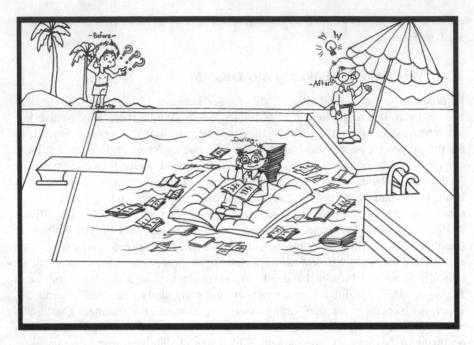

FIGURE 1.1 Swimming pool: Perspectives of 'immersion' and 'emergence' within the literature.

2   *The term originality is helpful to ensure that prospective researchers are aware that their research does not replicate the work of others.*
3   *The research should change the way we think about something, offer a paradigm/cultural shift by uncovering information that was previously underexplored or unknown.*

Whilst the aforementioned are important, it is also pertinent to highlight that some research may go against our cultural norm of a discipline. For instance, within the field of sociology, there is the assumption that researchers uncovering information that demonstrates poor practices, for instance, may lead to feelings of alienation or separation amongst peers (Coffey, 1999). The idea, then, of gaining acceptance is something a new researcher may need to contend with if/when deciding to embark on a specific field of interest (ibid). Little is written within the radiographic literature that accounts for such speculation, but prospective researchers are encouraged to reflect on potential feelings of alienation and/or events that may be deemed sensitive or hostile (Hayre and Hackett, 2020). Emotion is rarely discussed or considered as part of radiographic theses, perhaps linked to the view that emotion is epistemologically irrelevant (Barton and Reynold, 2003, p.100). Yet, in order for prospective researchers to understand both joy and difficulties experienced when undertaking research, it is argued here that it may become increasingly important that emotional reflections are provided and recognized as emotional virtue, rather than an emotional insignificance.

1.3.1 QUANTITATIVE RESEARCH

Quantitative researchers generally seek quantification of their findings, using numbers for breadth in what is often termed 'generalization' (Saks and Allsop, 2010). This is commonplace in experimental research, for instance, in diagnostic radiography, which the author(s) has utilized (Hayre et al., 2018; Mercardo and Hayre, 2018; Hayre, Jeffery and Bungay, 2020). In quantitative research, we often want to quantify X-ray photons, reaching radiosensitive organs, for instance. Here, researchers are primarily interested in variables whilst using calibrated instruments to demonstrate cause and effect relationships and identify ways of limiting ionizing radiation to phantoms.

Quantitative research has generally been more prominent in radiography when compared to its qualitative counterpart. This is unsurprising in light of its close affiliation with medicine and need for understanding the natural sciences associated with X-ray production and dose optimization. In the past, medical doctors were typically involved in performing X-rays and there are some excellent examples of this in early 20th century literature (Burrows, 1986). This symbiotic relationship between medicine and radiography still remains today in terms of the importance of quantifying and managing ionizing radiation and/or role extension by means of image interpretation. This naturally presents a strong rationale to perform quantitative research. Further, because radiography utilizes X-rays, a form of light eluding our senses, the need for objectivity and experimental research remains central by ensuring that its use is optimally applied. Arguably, then, diagnostic radiography remains closely aligned to positivism (discussed more in chapter 2), but there is also growing appreciation and contribution of qualitative research in our discipline. Whilst important, the application and understanding of quantitative approaches will remain paramount for undergraduate radiography students within undergraduate degree programmes. This will sustain theoretical knowledge and practice application, such as the quantification and limitation of scattered X-ray photons to both patients and staff. This often requires descriptive and inferential statistical analysis in order to support or enhance this new knowledge. Chapters 5–7 address the value and importance of quantitative approaches by providing the reader with applicable understandings, both methodologically and empirically.

1.3.2 QUALITATIVE RESEARCH

Qualitative research, on the other hand, is becoming increasingly used and relied upon within the field of diagnostic radiography. Whilst appreciated to remain polarized with quantitative work whereby empiricism is sought via non-numerical means, it can involve the use of field notes, transcripts, documents, pictures, diaries, audio notes and/or video recordings. The use of qualitative methods helps us understand the social practices, behaviours and attitudes of radiographic practitioners, for example. In my own doctorate study, qualitative approaches remained critical in observing 'what took place' during general imaging examinations (Hayre, 2016; Hayre et al., 2019). This is important because historically diagnostic radiography focused upon dose optimization using scientific and technical components of our practice with an underlying assumption that evidence is applied in everyday practice. Qualitative research may be overt or covert but primary focuses on uncovering phenomenon in-depth, when compared to its quantitative counterpart, which focuses on breadth. It is also important to recognize that qualitative research does not seek to resemble or replace quantitative approaches, it simply offers a perspective (or lens) that enables a researcher to explore phenomena that cannot (and perhaps, should not) be quantified, nor generalized. Further, because it does not seek generalization it does not mean it is less important. For instance, generalization may simply be improbable due to the phenomena understudied and/or whether it is too sensitive, or too limited, negating the possibility of external generalizability. It is, however, fair to assume that a clear distinction between qualitative and quantitative research exists and arguably essential in order to capture alternate data depending on the proposed research questions. There is also a more sinister view whereby individuals view one approach as superior to another. As an academic, it is not uncommon to hear colleagues advocating for quantitative research, considering it superior to qualitative approaches. A general theme in this book is an overarching appreciation of each methodological approach, which is driven by the projects aim and questions of an intended study.

For students reading this text, we have an opportunity to learn and appreciate the value of each research paradigm, whilst considering their respective merits without conforming to pessimism. Further discussions around the rationale and application of qualitative research can be found in chapters 8–10, whereby methodological strategies, methods, data analysis and trustworthiness are discussed providing a lens on the utility of qualitative work and how it can be approached by prospective researchers.

1.4   THREE P'S TO ENGAGING IN THE RESEARCH PROCESS

Acknowledgment of maintaining an overarching goal is important, for which the 'three p's' are introduced – preparing, participating and probing. For preparation, we consider this stage as laying the foundations of an intended study, such as, obtaining relevant knowledge pertinent to the research – what we currently know in the paradigm. This will involve reading and drawing from a wide range of sources. This appraisal of the literature is important to see if the proposed work has been repeated or whether it remains worthwhile. The underpinning philosophy is also central when engaging in this process and thus recommended. Chapter 2 examines varying philosophies and also how our philosophical assumptions are tested or altered, especially for those engaging in doctorate research. Upon reflection of our philosophical assumptions, it is recommended that researchers do not assume a philosophical lens. Quite the contrary, this is an intriguing and rewarding part of any research process whereby engagement and scholarly debate leads to alternate discourses. As acknowledged, this phase of the research does not need an immediate decision as it may evolve and also alter the direction of a study in order to meet the intended goals. Other important features are associated with preparing and developing the aim(s), objectives and/or research questions. Finally, and perhaps more importantly, prior to engaging in the 'participating' phase, researchers should now have a sound methodological plan, accompanied with ethical tools and approvals facilitating the undertaking of an intended study – chapters 3 and 4 assist new researchers in this phase.

Preparation enables researchers to get 'as close as reasonably possible' to participate in order to satisfy submission to an ethics committee. The participation stage, however, which is linked to the collection of empirical data (regardless of the research strategy employed). If experimental, this may involve going into an X-ray room and performing predetermined X-ray exposures using a phantom and dosimeter. On the other hand, it may involve the researcher 'participating' in observations, interviews and/or focus groups, for instance. At this stage, we accept that researchers may be required to adjust or adapt in response to unexpected findings. Here, the concept of reflexivity may be put into practice. For qualitative researchers, however, the process is more complex because researchers remain the key instrument throughout the data collection phase, which interconnects with the data analysis. In chapters 9, 10 and 11, the practice of reflexivity [and positionality] are detailed to demonstrate the significance of researcher participation, but also his/her influences on the qualitative research process itself. The final 'p' is 'probing'. Here, we can consider this as the third stage of a research process whereby the collection of empiricism has now ceased. At this point, it is now the role of the researcher to probe (or push), via critical analysis, and evaluate, with a focus on uncovering original empiricism. The ability to probe and write with intent remains essential in order to not only add to the existing evidence, but offer impactful outcomes, coupled with good storytelling. In short, the need for 'probing' or 'pushing' out from our confined boundaries helps develop current ways of thinking and perhaps doing. It is essential not only for dissertation and thesis writing, but also for academic dissemination, in either peer-reviewed journals or other scholarly outputs.

1.5 CONTEMPORARY CONTEXT FOR RADIOGRAPHY RESEARCH

Let's first imagine a world without research in radiography and our inability to advance knowledge. This lack of critical appraisal and openness to challenge would naturally put our patients at risk. We have identified the plethora of evidence that informs dose optimization upon the utilization of radiation or understanding interests and needs of service users. When considering our research in radiography, we should be reminded that it does not seek to benefit ourselves, but our patients. Radiography is person-centred and patients will remain at the forefront of healthcare delivery and research. If we fail to engage or continue on our research journey, it is likely to prevent us from thinking about what we do, how we do it and seek change for positive outcomes. Arguably, then, our professional practice and knowledge would become stagnant, trapped in a doctrine of old schools of thought and prevented from developing radiological diagnosis, safety and care.

The number of radiographers participating in research remains generally small. This is unsurprising owing to the vocational nature of our profession and likelihood of graduates progressing and continuing into clinical roles, rather than research roles. However, radiography has a growing research culture, which will naturally increase as our demand for evidence based continues. This has the potential for creating a research focused role in radiography for those finding a balance between practice and research. Specifically, a number of dedicated journals are enhancing the research culture and uncovering various forms of research on the qualitative and quantitative spectrum. This is critical. The outlook for radiography research, then, is positive and perhaps safe to assume that radiography research is excelling, with anticipation it remains sustainable. Current and future challenges associated with radiography research not only concerns its implementation, but also its attractiveness. Whilst a divide between what is practiced in accordance with the evidence-based literature exists, this will require greater consideration, with perhaps the emergence of new roles. In previous works, the role of 'Digital Radiography Champion' has been proffered, for instance (Hayre and Cox, 2020). Here, the idea accepts that general radiography is ever-changing, whether technological, dose related or patient centric, thus the 'Champion' role would act as a conduit between research and practice in order to transfer evidence in a systematic, yet auditable way.

Our engagement in research, as a profession has also enabled us to critically examine and reshape healthcare delivery. Whilst a research focus continues to be supported with professional bodies and regarded as a core feature for both undergraduate and postgraduate education, there is some insight that research may not always remain a core feature for all graduating healthcare professionals. For example, experiences working in Australia have led to discussions surrounding the cessation of 'Research Methods' as an undergraduate subject for radiography students. Further, upon comparison with the United Kingdom, for instance, graduates from Australia may not always graduate with honours. For students in some higher education institutions wishing to engage in 'honours work/research', it is considered additional academic activity, which requires to be engagement outside their exisiting undergraduate programme. The potential cessation of research methods within the curriculum identifes that it may not remain an essential subject for teaching and learning for medical radiation practitioners, in Australia. This is not widespread but arguably detrimental in future years whereby radiographers lack basic research skills upon entering the clinical setting and upon engaging with the evidence based as part of their own continuous professional development. Further, it is likely to limit the virtues and challenges of research methods, coupled with interpreting empirical evidence. This is important to reflect upon if research subjects become obsolete for some and not for others, arguably questioning parity of radiography graduates.

Reasons for ensuring that research is sustained within our profession is threefold. First, for us to remain critical thinkers, radiographers (and educators) must be accustomed to methodological processes. For instance, being able to identify originality within a specific field, not only identifies potential for change within the clinical setting, but also challenges the status quo, removing dogmatic views that assert 'it has always been done this way'. By enriching the student radiographer, practitioner or prospective researcher with a 'can do' attitude, it can instil a philosophy that considers radiographic evidence as paramount. Second, there is a general acceptance (and danger) that practitioners may become increasingly complacent in the everyday doctrine of medical imaging thus important for researchers to continuously challenge, explore and solve issues within our clinical environments. In chapter 2, a discussion pertaining to postmodernism seeks to prevent such practices by dispelling ideas that have perhaps linguistically been coerced overtime. By conforming, this may give rise to alternate practices or cultures that become toxic or simply fail to critically evaluate what they do, how they do it and how to improve. Third, the process of knowing and understanding how research fits into the radiography environment is important, but, there are other components to radiography research that evolve as researchers move into uncomfortable spaces. For instance, engaging in research philosophy can not only provide a deepened awareness of philosophical thought, but also facilitates thought-provoking concepts, such as whether it is time to destabilize and deconstruct what we have come to know (postmodernism) or simply understand diversity in behaviour and attitudes (interpretivism). These modes of thinking were not on my 'tick list' when deciding to embark onto a PhD, but are considered in my academic writing, research and teaching. In short, the landscape of research in radiography is positive as evidence continues to grow worldwide. The examination of multiple facets previously underexplored clearly demonstrates a more open and critical dialogue into radiographic practices. This offers a clear advantage. However, there is a potential pitfall, as noted above whereby some students, and subsequent practitioners may lack 'research exposure' when compared to others during their undergraduate studies. Does this disadvantage them or disadvantage the patients in their care? Probably both. What can be accepted is that the interpretation of a 'graduating radiographer' may depend on his or her place of education and geography thus mindful of the future workforces and educational differences for future graduates understanding research in radiography.

1.6 CHAPTER SUMMARY

This chapter sought to provide an introductory perspective to readers embarking into radiography research for the first time. The chapter began by situating research in the radiography context, whilst asserting what it offers. It was then important to identify (and introduce) some important terms and concepts, such as originality and paradigms. From experience, it has been found that a strong understanding of terms has enabled dissertation students, for instance, to grapple with the importance of not only undertaking research in radiography, but ensuring it offers new and insightful knowledge. Next, the introduction of preparing, participating and probing is noted as an overarching strategy encapsulating the research process as a whole, especially in its early stages. Such foresight is important because it enables prospective researchers to understand expectations of the research journey when embarking on a research project for the first time. Lastly, recognition and some debate concerning radiography research in the contemporary space is added. This not only celebrates the value of research practice in our profession, but also acknowledges the challenges of implementing research evidence into the everyday clinical context, whilst also raising questions around epistemological differences.

KEY TERMS

Empiricism: theory that knowledge is derived from the senses and an umbrella term for research emanating from quantitative and qualitative research.
Epistemological theory: is concerned with the study and nature of knowledge and aligned to a core facet of philosophy.

Evidence base: is based on the idea that empirically published works are used to inform occupational practices.

Generalization: is regarded as a general statement or concept obtained by inference from specific X-ray experiments, for example.

Methodology: is a contextual framework for research, a logical approach to answering research questions and guided by the researchers' values, beliefs and systems of knowing.

Narrative: is a spoken or written account of connected events, such as an interview transcript or referenced in storytelling.

Natural Sciences: is a branch of science that deals with the physical world, such as X-rays.

Originality: is termed as having the ability to think independently and creatively and thus linked to the creation of new knowledge.

Paradigm: a distinct set of ideas or concepts, which may involve theories, research methods, and radiography standards that are generally accepted within the field.

Paradigm shift: is a fundamental change in the basic concepts and practices of a discipline, i.e., the change to a commonly held perspective of a radiographic technique.

Qualitative: research that relies on data obtained by researchers utilizing methods such as participant observation, interviewing, focus groups and documentation.

Quantitative: research that seeks to quantify data amongst researchers and typically linked with surveys and X-ray laboratory experiments in radiography research.

Reflexive/Reflexivity: linked to sociology and is principally references to a circular relationship between interactions and effects embedded in human beliefs, actions and behaviours.

Social actors: are considered those individuals that can help shape a particular ideology or discourse pertinent to a particular event.

Social sciences: is devoted to the study of a society and any relationships shared amongst a particular group within that society.

EXERCISES AND STUDY QUESTIONS

1   Consider what research means for the radiography profession? In your answer, think about the opportunities and challenges that will arise as we accept and participate in research practices for enhancing our everyday knowledge.

2   When thinking about quantitative and qualitative research, discern the differences between the two, from both a theoretical and practical standpoint.

3   Upon examination of the research process as a whole, reflect on the three central tenets above and how these allow you to navigate your own prospective research journey.

REFERENCES

Adams, R., (1975) "Where Do Our Ideas Come From? Descartes vs Locke", reprinted in Stitch S. (Ed.) Innate Ideas, Berkeley, CA: California University Press.

Barton, C. and Reynold E. (2003) 'Dilemmas of control'. In R. Lee and E. Stanko (Eds.) *Researching Violence: Essays on Methodology and Measurement.* London: Routledge, pp. 88–106.

Burrows, E. H. (1986) *Pioneers and Early Years of British Radiology*. Hampshire: Colophan.

Coffey, A. (1999) *The Ethnographic Self.* London: Sage.

Griffiths, P, and Norman, I. (2013) 'Qualitative or quantitative? Developing and evaluating complex interventions: time to end the paradigm war'. *International Journal of Nursing Studies,* 50 (5), pp. 583–584.

Hammersley, M. and Atkinson, P. (2007) *Ethnography Principles in Practice,* 3rd Edn, New York: Routledge.

Hayre, C.M. (2016) 'Cranking up', 'whacking up' and 'bumping up': X-ray exposures in contemporary radiographic practice. *Radiography*, 22 (2), pp. 194–198.

Hayre, C.M., Blackman, S., Carlton, K. and Eyden, A. (2019) The use of cropping and digital side markers (DSM) in digital radiography. *Journal of Medical Imaging and Radiation Sciences*, 50 (2), pp. 234–242.

Hayre, C.M., Bungay, H., Jeffery, C., Cobb, C., and Atutornu, J. (2018) Can placing lead-rubber inferolateral to the light beam diaphragm limit ionising radiation to multiple radiosensitive organs? *Radiography.* 24 (1), pp. 15–21.

Hayre, C.M. and Cox, W.A.S.C. (2020) *General Radiography Principles and Practices.* Boca Raton: CRC Press.

Hayre, C.M. and Hackett, P.M.W. (2020) *Handbook of Ethnography in Healthcare Research.* New York: Routledge.

Hayre, C.M. Jeffery, C., and Bungay, H. (2020) Do lead-rubber aprons always limit ionising radiation to radiosensitive organs? *Radiography,* 26 (4), pp. e264–e269.

Kuhn, T.S. (1962) *The Structure of Scientific Revolutions,* Chicago: The University of Chicago Press.

Mercardo, L. and Hayre, C.M. (2018) The detection of wooden foreign bodies: an experimental study comparing direct digital radiography (DDR) and ultrasonography. *Radiography,* 24 (3), pp. 340–344.

O'Reilly, K. (2011) *Ethnographic Methods*, 2nd Edn, New York: Routledge.

Saks, M. and Allsop, J. (2010) *Researching Health, Qualitative, Quantitative and Mixed Methods*, London: Sage.

2 Philosophical Foundations for Radiography Research

Christopher M. Hayre

2.1 INTRODUCTION

This chapter introduces and explains philosophical principles and how these are intertwined in radiography research. Upon thinking about philosophy, we may not assume it clearly links with research *per se,* but it does. Not forgetting that if/when someone decides to embark onto a PhD, they are naturally studying and engaging in a doctorate of philosophy, thus understandings concerning philosophical constructs and emergence of alternate views and philosophical dispositions are important when it comes to understanding and appreciating the varied nature of philosophical thought. This chapter focuses on the generally accepted and less accepted views of philosophy for research purposes. This is important in order to help undergraduate and/or postgraduate students come to terms with ascertaining its rationality in terms of viewing the world around us, and thus how knowledge is generated. Two additional books are recommended here for emphasis on the philosophy of science (Couvalis, 1999) and the philosophy of social science (Benton and Craib, 2001).

This chapter discusses two important philosophical concepts – ontology and epistemology. In order for researchers to ground themselves in what they intend to examine, they should ask themselves how they 'see reality' [ontology] and ask how knowledge is generated [epistemology]. In my first PhD supervisory meeting I was tasked with examining my own ontology and epistemology. Researchers reading this book and looking to engage in research for the first time are also encouraged to critically examine their own ontology and epistemology in order to critique the research topic, which of course, may change. This chapter, then, is not only a reflective positional narrative, but also examines peer-reviewed work that seeks to challenge customary norms. This is important as this text is aimed at undergraduate students, thus whilst convention is important, it also seeks to offer an alternate approach, which can be applied in radiography and elsewhere. This is important as it may pave the way for alternate philosophical thinking that is both unique and fulfilling, leading to different methodological designs and later empiricism.

DOI: 10.1201/9780367559311-2

2.2   WHAT IS RESEARCH PHILOSOPHY?

If embarking onto a PhD, be mindful that you are participating in a 'doctorate of philosophy', not a 'doctorate of radiography'. You are, essentially, philosophizing about your research topic. When we think about philosophy, in general, it points to a specific set of beliefs and/or assumptions. For research, this is principally linked to the nature of our reality and development of knowledge, as a primary objective for many researchers and identified previously in chapter 1. Here, then, whether we accept it or not, we subconsciously align ourselves to a research philosophy. The purpose of this chapter is to uncover these philosophical models, but also provide insight for the reader that may align, offer clarification or opposition. Regardless of the outcome, researchers are encouraged to engage in this process, now and throughout the research, facilitating potential for wider philosophical debate in radiography. It may also further help develop unique or previously suppressed schools of thought in order to build on existing knowledge and understanding for future researchers.

Prior to delving into widely recognized principles, it is important to identify three key terms. First is ontology, which is associated with our reality around us and focuses on concepts of existence. For instance, there can be an ontology that is aligned to objectivism, also known as foundationalism, which accepts a single and immutable reality (Couvalis, 1999). On the other hand, social constructionism considers multiple realities that are continually reconstructed based on social actors (Benton and Craib, 2001). In short, ontology is concerned with how you 'see' your research. If seeking to optimize ionizing radiation, you are likely to be aligning to objectivism, whereas upon observing the behaviour of radiographers, the according ontology is aligned to social constructionism. Second is epistemology, and by using examples above, a clear link can be made. An 'epistemological position' reflects the view of what we can know about the world and how we can know it (Marsh and Furlong, 2002). For instance, if a researcher deems their ontology to be objectivist, they will usually have a similar positivist epistemology. Conversely, if social constructionism remains the researchers choice of ontology, then (s)he will have an according interpretivist epistemology (Weber, 1946, p.152). There is some appreciation that researchers may find themselves on either side of the philosophical spectrum. Sherman and Webb (1988, p.13) claim that the 'compatibility and the call for cooperation between qualitative and quantitative enquiry cannot be sustained since the two approaches come close to speaking different languages'. In response, for some researchers in distinct disciplines, this may be the case, but the position here seeks to reflect a complimentary appreciation of opposing ontologies and epistemologies for radiography research. The term 'epistemology' is derived from the Greek words *epistēmē* (knowledge) and *logos* (reason), hence the notion that it remains concerned with the theory of knowledge. Epistemology can be individualistic, leaning to what constitutes acceptability, validity and legitimacy. In radiography, we currently accept various forms of knowledge generation and is represented within respected journals worldwide. Within the radiographic space, the first author's research clearly offers a juxtaposed perspective whereby his involvement in research spans across opposing epistemologies – positivism

(Hayre, Bungay and Jerrey, 2020) and interpretivism (Benfield et al., in press). But, for other disciplines, such as medicine, there is growing debate that perhaps favours one school of thought over another (Loder, 2016). This demonstrates that differences may not always lead to acceptance, nor do all epistemological views resonate with particular disciplines. Whilst it is beyond the scope of this chapter to critically examine this here, recent outputs concerning the unification of qualitative and quantitative methods in health, rehabilitation and medicine in the authors own work can be found (Hayre and Blackman, 2020; Hayre et al., in press).

Third is axiology and refers to the values and ethics within our research. For instance, as researchers, we may hold strong views about a particular area of radiographic practice, or have, ourselves undergone a particular experience, which may drive our research agenda. In my work, the decision to examine the impact of digital radiography equipment in the clinical environment was in response to observations and reflections as both a radiography student, and then, a radiographic practitioner (Hayre, 2016a). Looking back, the key driver for pursuing a PhD was based on the practice of radiographers using X-ray exposures, comforting patients, which coincided with overt challenges relating to knowledge and understanding of new equipment (ibid). By highlighting this, it asserts that our own values guide reason and action in the research space. In practice, this remains commonplace, observing researchers favouring topics, say, in magnetic resonance imaging (MRI), computed tomography (CT) imaging or general imaging (as I did). Thus, in relation to the axiology in our research, exploring the general imaging environment, rather than a specialism, was grounded by the premise that general radiography consists of approximately 80% of all imaging examinations performed in the clinical environment. Henceforth, the intention was to explore an imaging modality that remained a large portion of what we do as radiographers, which also anticipated links to other image modalities. In short, there is perhaps an onus on ensuring any chosen topic remains of interest as it will be linked to your values and beliefs that eventually drive you to completion. Here, prospective researchers (on all philosophical spectrums) are encouraged to document their axiology upon undertaking research in order to help build an emotional connection (or even resilience) with the desired topic, whilst underscoring the rationale for undertaking your desired research in the first place.

The abovementioned philosophical queries and virtues can guide researchers in research design, data collection and data analysis, depending on the research agenda. Looking back on the axiology in my research, there was a philosophical process of succumbing to conventional thought processes by reflecting on previous experiences, either professionally or personally. In order to break out of this conventional space, researchers should adopt a reflexive skill set throughout the research process, whilst mindful of initial thought processes. Further, by positioning our underlying philosophies to reality, knowledge and values, it is important to consider that this may be later refined or redesigned as we continue throughout. The key, for any early staged student or practitioner, is to not only engage with the literature surrounding the area of interest, but remain open minded and not always conform to specific perspectives or doctrines previously held.

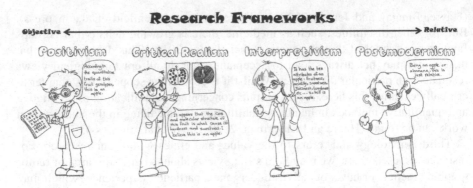

FIGURE 2.1 Epistemological frameworks for Radiographic Researchers.

Is there a quick fix, you may ask? For some, little attention concerning this process may prevail, which has often been heard as: 'we're positivists and always will be!'. This, for some experimentalists may offer a quick and easy solution for researchers performing experimental research. On the other hand, there is an argument of losing an opportunity to intellectually immerse oneself within the philosophical realms of research, which offers alternate possibilities for engaging in, say, less practiced philosophies, such as critical realism or postmodernism? The latter may offer reform in the search for an applied evidence based by deconstructing or destabilizing contemporary thought processes and help bridge an evidence–practice gap. There are two terms that can help contextualize our schools of thought when it comes to approaching the spectrum of philosophical theory. First, the term unificationist, which observes radiographic research as fragmented whereby alternate approaches (such as critical realism, interpretivism or postmodernism) are somehow watering down or diluting the true scientific nature of our research. The unificationist would concede that radiography research should fall under one philosophy, one paradigmatic thinking and thus one according methodology (DiFrisco, 2019). The term pluralist, on the other hand, accepts diversity within the philosophical context whilst seeking alternate forms of knowledge development. If we examine radiography practice, we see that pluralism examines the varied nature of people/patients, a culture or its practices that take place within our profession, as represented by Figure 2.1. It not only allows for alternate philosophical thought, but seeks to address diverse outlooks within our professional space. Here, researchers may welcome the pluralist's point of view, which, in my view reflects the varying nature and practice of our profession now and in years to come.

2.3 PHILOSOPHY OF EXPERIMENTAL RESEARCHERS

When we think about underpinning philosophies linking experimental research in radiography, objectivism is likely to remain our primary ontological position. As an author to several experimental papers, conforming to this philosophical approach is important, yet not formally reported. As an objectivist, we are empirically affiliating ourselves with the natural sciences – X-ray photons. Because of our need to opti-mize X-rays clinical, there is naturally a need to apply an objectivist ontology and an according positivist epistemology. Here, the term positivism is used, but there have been further developments since its inception, i.e., radical positivism, Comtean positivism, logical positivism and post-positivism. For the purpose and scope of this chapter, in particular with reference to critical realism, interpretivism and postmod-ernism, the collective term positivism will be used.

Auguste Comte is regarded as the first philosopher of science outlining three stages in the quest for truth and achievement of positivism (theological, metaphys-ical and the positive). Whilst the term 'positivism' is recognized and accepted when it comes to offering philosophical commentaries (Hayre et al., in press), we should not dismiss latter movements of logical positivism and post-positivism, as additions. For instance, the former affirms that other than the empirical evidence itself, logical thought processes remain an important source of knowledge development. The latter, post-positivism, argues that all forms of observation lead to some form of error (Denzin, 1997). In light of these recent philosophies, we are now in a position to accept that the pursuit of 'truth' in experimental research is problematic and thus positivists only seek to get as close to the truth as possible, vis-à-vis, post-positivism (ibid).

Positivism is principally positioned within the natural sciences, which provides sound reasoning for adopting it as a theory of knowledge. In addition, it is also central for the development of current evidence. For instance, radiographers around the world work closely with X-ray photons, producing ionizing radiation, which cannot be seen, heard or felt. Yet, radiographers are required to produce, cease and optimize it within their everyday work. Positivists are seeking to create law-like generalizations, and although the term 'proof' and 'truth' are not accepted, positivism aims to uncover sci-entific knowledge that is as accurate as possible in order to facilitate medical imaging practices. Clearly, the need for experimental research in radiography is paramount, and will continue to remain paramount in order for us to both understand and opti-mize this form of light, which eludes our human senses.

This clearly strengthens our rationale for considering positivism whilst performing experimental research, whereby the radiographic community learns and develops from empiricism that influences decision making and helps drive national or inter-national policy. As seen in Figure 2.2, when observing an apple, positivism seeks to identify phenomena in both the natural and scientific world, in its objective form.

The value of quantitative research will importantly remain commonplace for practitioners transnationally in order to help limit, but also optimize this hazard within our profession. In radiography, it is clear that our need for experimental research, driven by positivism is essential for both the foundation and continued evi-dence in order for the profession to learn, deliver and sustain excellence in radio-graphic imaging. A clear distinction closely affiliated with positivism is hypothetical deduction, which aims to reduce the author's experience and theory to a specified experimental method(s), involving independent and dependent variables prior to undertaking the experiment (Sheppard, 2007). Thus, when we come to think about philosophical principles aligned to such hypothetical-deductive reasoning, we are naturally drawn to positivism, vis-à-vis the scientific experimental model.

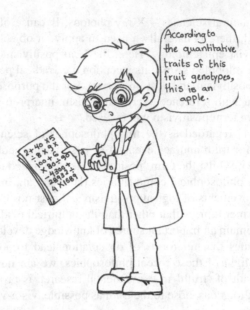

FIGURE 2.2   A positivist lens of examining an apple.

As noted above, this philosophy is expressed by its exclusivity in which it focuses on the natural sciences, i.e., those closely associated with the natural phenomena; it is claimed that both reason and logic are inferred and remain an exclusive source of all certain knowledge. We have already proffered the claim that positivist data are deemed 'factual' by demonstrating 'proof', as data conforms to the natural laws in our everyday society (Pole and Morrison, 2003). Here, then, if you decide to undertake an X-ray experiment, it would be sensible to assume that your philosophical underpinning will align to positivism, coupled with an ontology of objectivism. My view is that whilst the traditional view of positivism within the radiographic community is still accepted, for new and prospective researchers, critical evaluation is still recommended in accordance with logical positivism and/or post-positivism.

In addition to positivism, researchers may find solace by moving further along the philosophical spectrum, whereby 'critical realism' can be met. Before this is explored, it is important to discern 'critical realism' from 'realism'. The latter closely resembles affiliation with an individual or any given object in reality, remaining objective. As you have already imagined, this closely resembles the world of positivism, but involves individuals or objects. Critical realism has been previously considered as the conduit between positivism and post-positivism, whereas critical realists view their ontology as the same (by means of independence of a single reality) and distanced by means of maintaining objectivity, but may still come up with different assumptions (Pole and Morrison, 2003). This can be seen in Figure 2.3 using our analogy of the apple.

Another significant difference with critical realism is the examination of experiences of those individuals of a professional group. For instance, then, a researcher may wish to understand and perform a particular X-ray experiment in order to seek some novelty. Yet, whilst a radiographer may wish to undertake an X-ray experiment, establishing

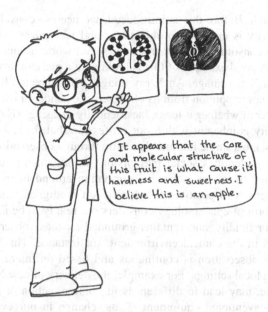

FIGURE 2.3 A critical realist lens of observing an apple.

conditions to create the experimental model and then observe their results, a critical realist would argue that the results are caused by underlying theoretical mechanisms, structures and laws that they cannot observe (Haigh et al., 2019). In this situation, unlike most other philosophies, the ontology and epistemology are separate, whereas typically, they are interlinked.

Another analogy that can be linked to critical realism in our everyday practice is the detection of pathology. For instance, on the one hand, a radiologist (who perhaps considers themselves as a realist) would say, based on his/her decision-making will rationalize their diagnosis affirming, 'I identify pathology as I see it!' Contrary to this, a radiologist leaning towards a critical realist position would argue that the 'realist radiologist' may only have observed one aspect of the pathology. For example, could the positioning of the patient be a factor that either facilitates or hinders the diagnosis? This analogy helps us because whilst both radiologists would agree that the patient and radiograph remain objective, neither radiologist has observed the imaging take place. Thus, whilst the ontology of the radiologists remains the same, their epistemologies (how they come up with knowledge – the diagnosis) are different and are thus alternately constructed based on their observations. It is this sensory data by radiologists that requires justification in our reasoning, upon which a diagnosis is made.

2.4 PHILOSOPHY OF NATURALISTIC RESEARCHERS

At this point, we have moved further 'right' on our philosophical spectrum. We began with positivism, on the far left. Then, shifting further right, we acknowledge critical realism. Moving along the spectrum even further we arrive at naturalistic enquiries to research. Before this is introduced, we need to consider the term sub-jectivity. Subjectivity is opposed to objectivity and recognizes the experiences of those people who constitute and construct the social world around them (Pole and Morrison, 2003). A good example of this is looking at a piece of artwork, a painting, for instance, or an X-ray image. An X-ray image, whilst created by scientific tools may draw differences in opinion from its observers, i.e., under or overexposure, over-rotation and/or overall whether it looks 'aesthetically pleasing' (Hayre et al., 2019). Clearly, subjectivity is inherent within our profession, but for researchers, subject-ivism does not assume a single immutable reality through observation (unlike object-ivism). Subjectivity identifies social participants, informants or actors that remain part of a group and to whom interpret information around them (Denzin, 1997). If objectivism aligns with positivism, subjectivism is aligned with interpretivism. Remember, this form of epistemology considers our reality to be in a constant state of revision, flux or fluidity, and remains grounded by those observing and acting, like radiographers in the clinical environment, for instance. This remodelling and reconstructing via observation is continuous and based on interactions with peers and objects within local settings. For example, the delivery of new X-ray equipment, a symbolic feature, may lead to differences in opinion, action or behaviour, when compared with conventional equipment. Thus, change in our everyday contexts, whether X-ray equipment or staffing can alter the behaviour of individuals and argu-ably lead to alternate radiographic realities. Whilst this remains of interest to qualita-tive researchers, it also prevents qualitative researchers from generalizing empirical findings. Whilst low sampling may be deemed problematic, it arguably reflects the ever-changing and evolving or limited number of events affiliated with naturalistic events (Saks and Allsop, 2010). Thus in radiography research, the complex nature of differing opinions, cultures, clinical environments and attitudes play a key role when it comes to evaluating empiricism within the naturalistic space.

Upon discussing philosophies pertinent to naturalistic events, we need to acknow-ledge the juxtaposed framework in which naturalistic research sits, especially when compared with experimental models. For instance, experimental researchers aim to delineate thought-provoking assumptions of the social world and develop experiments that remain distanced from researchers. This objective state is achieved by separating the researcher with his/her experiment (although as we have already alluded, our axiology may guide the researcher). On the other hand, however, for the naturalist researcher, their goal is exploration of subjective experiences within the natural envir-onment. For instance, the naturalistic researcher utilizes their own subjective experi-ence in order to explore the environment and participants of interest. The definition of the natural environment is associated with the practice in which it is carried out, i.e., general radiography, CT and/or theatre radiography. One obvious example is the author's own naturalistic enquiry exploring the practices of diagnostic radiographers using digital radiography equipment (Hayre, 2016a). For this naturalistic inquest, its intention sought to capture individual experiences and interactions of phenomena pertinent to the researcher's interests (ibid).

As we move 'further right' along our epistemological spectrum, our interests move into the subjective realms of interpretivism. Whilst it is not 'the end' of our spectrum, interpretivism is generally accepted to be opposed to positivism. It accepts that knowledge collated from individuals cannot be linked to any physical phenomena, which occur in the natural world, i.e., X-ray photons. For interpretivist researchers, then, the principle goal is perhaps observing or engaging in knowledge generation that uncovers behaviours of individuals, with a primary objective of uncovering both description and depth, rather than breadth. In Figure 2.4 descriptors seek to identify the apple by using the individuals human senses, attributing its 'sweetness', 'toughness' and 'juiciness' in this case. This, from an interpretivist view may differ with another individual's interpretation of the apple, as such, someone that perhaps dislikes the taste or appearance of apples.

Unlike the perspective of positivists (or realists), interpretivists recognize that not all individuals behave in 'law-abiding' patterns, but recognize that individuals may often have deep-rooted feelings behind their actions, behaviours or attitudes (Saks and Allsop, 2010). For instance, whilst we may consider radiography and X-ray exposure selection as a 'scientific practice', the nature of X-ray exposure selection/manipulation itself remains a subjective form of practice, as radiographers observe a patient, body habitus and suspected pathology under investigation, later selecting an appropriate exposure based on feeling or intuition. This offers a subjective component to our radiographic practice, which has now been recognized. The example of X-ray exposure manipulation amongst radiographers, for example, now offers evidence demonstrating both unknowing and knowing awareness to increases in ionizing radiation to patients (Hayre, 2016b). The rationale, by radiographers, was based on a radiographer's belief or attitude concerning image quality. Here, we can see

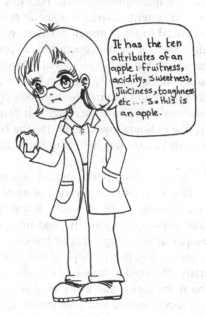

FIGURE 2.4 An interpretivist's lens of observing the apple.

that whilst it may be assumed that radiographers apply scientific reasoning (perhaps hypothetically deductive) in terms of exposure factor selection, this is not always the case and further supports the increasing need for qualitative research whereby assumptions of current practice are generally developed via positivist models, which are assumed to be applied. In addition, there is an increasing disconnect between what is experimented scientifically, with (and evidenced) what is practiced and applied in the everyday setting.

Interpretivism, then, allows a researcher to build alternate knowledge in diagnostic radiography by remaining affiliated with subjectivism. Interpretivism may also be known as 'anti-positivism', 'anti-naturalism' or 'anti-foundationalism', as indicated by its opposition above, but has a common goal – to uncover individualist summaries or constructions concerning the interpretation of the social world around them (Sheppard, 2007). Further, whereas deduction is a form of reasoning used in X-ray experiments to refine and hypothetically examine theory in attempts to falsify, naturalistic research requires inductive reasoning in order to 'build-up' novel epistemology previously uncaptured. This is important because researchers that hold interpretivist views typically believe that research on human beings, by human beings, cannot yield objective results (Denzin, 1997). This leads to an accumulation and identification of subjective experiences of individuals engaging in a specific social interaction. In my work and upon the exploration of day-to-day radiography practices with diagnostic radiographers, immersion amongst radiographers (as a radiographer myself) remained essential in order to generate new knowledge from the bottom-up. Because this topic remained unique in the radiography community, it anticipated to generate theoretical knowledge for that community. This form of philosophical reasoning, then, is naturally affiliated with qualitative methods, later discussed in chapter 8.

For qualitative researchers, interpretivism and social constructionism arguably remain the 'go to' philosophical forms of enquiry. These ontological and epistemological schools of thought have enabled the generation of previously undocumented knowledge, which has not only led to the development of larger research designs, but also helped influence policy transnationally (British Institute of Radiology, 2020). It is my view that research involving naturalistic methods does, and will, continue to impact and develop the profession in future years. It can enable members of a professional community, like radiography, to examine the behaviours, actions and attitudes of its members, whilst assisting with the application of evidence-based radiography.

Readers embarking onto their own philosophical journeys for the first time would be right to assume that interpretivism (in light of its opposition to positivism) completes the philosophical spectrum from which researchers may seek to use. However, another essential philosophy moves beyond interpretivism (and thus further right) on our philosophical spectrum. This is known as postmodernism. This branch of underpinning philosophy moves beyond our critique of positivism and objectivism and is generally attributed to linguistics (Holliday, 2016). A key feature of postmodernist thinking is the notion that everything is continuously in a state of change, such as the X-ray environment, and that knowledge generation features a fluid state. Because postmodernists accept that language remains a cause that brings

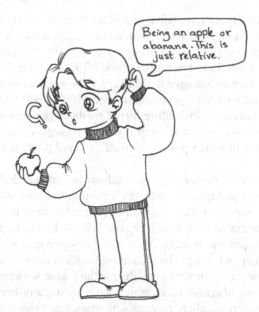

FIGURE 2.5   The postmodernist view of the apple.

about change, it is also recognized that language has the potential to oppress and/or exclude ideas within a particular field (ibid), perhaps the X-ray or academic environment, for instance? As seen in Figure 2.5, the postmodernist may not be concerned with what the apple was, but concerned with how it is understood.

It is argued that because our social and radiographic 'order' has been derived from language over many years, it is difficult to ascertain whether our language is, now, appropriate. This, in turn, leads to a critique that radiography has been shaped by language and grounded on the medical model of positivism. It can be assumed that if positivism is and continues to be interconnected with the constructs of radiographic epistemology, this will resonate in our everyday narrative and language of the actors involved. Importantly, however, it does not suppose that this is correct, but simply a perspective that fits to a moment in time amongst its members. It is important to note that if you are seeking to perform or rationalize postmodernism as a research philosophy, it could arguably be considered as a school of thought which has been largely suppressed, when compared to previously mentioned epistemological counterparts. On an optimistic note, potential awaits for the utilization and application of postmodernism by offering new ways in thinking, doing or researching in radiography. If our linguistic modes can be challenged, strengthened or distanced, this may facilitate our development in knowledge.

Thinking as a postmodern researcher, a key role will be to seek and expose dogmatic schools of thought, thus requiring a form of 'deconstruction', 'disestablishing' or 'knocking down and rebuilding' in order to search for frailties within widely held truths (Kilduff and Mehra, 1997). An example, which hints of a postmodern-radiographic turn has been captured by Holliday (2016) recognizing how the deconstruction of observing qualitative and quantitative methods as mutual (Hayre, 2016a) offered a postmodern way of conducting research in radiography. Simply, the decision not to conform, yet, apply a perspective that affirmed qualitative and quantitative research as a whole and not mixed (ibid). That said, for the purposes of this book, whilst readers are encouraged to think critically when it comes to destabilizing conventions, especially within a postmodern space, it is important for undergraduate purposes that our narrative surrounding mixed methods remains in some part, conventional. This, however, does not mean it cannot be argued against, nor hinted of alternate possibilities in which postmodernism can, and perhaps should, be applied in some instances.

For those undertaking higher degrees, students are encouraged to examine their research philosophies and question whether a postmodern lens would help enhance not only empirical originality, but also methodological novelty in a given study. One other challenge associated with this, however, will be linked to dissemination and acceptance amongst peers as it seeks to question our status quo or shed light on alternate ways of knowing and doing. The goal of postmodern thinking is perhaps, in part, suggesting some form of radical change, dismantling what we know, and have come to know by providing alternate ideas which have historically been suppressed. By engaging in this way, researchers emerge with empirical evidence that is unique or perhaps historically excluded/muted, but in return, it also requires some philosophical acceptance at least, especially to strongly held perspectives or beliefs. In these situations, it will be important to reflect on power relationships because whilst power relations cannot be avoided, researchers need to be content with their spiritual, ethical and/or moral dispositions in order to critically think and engage with the language and practices in which postmodernism applies.

2.5 PHILOSOPHY FOR MIXED METHOD RESEARCHERS

Upon reflection and overtime, I have developed an appreciation for qualitative and quantitative techniques. In my view, the value of experimental papers, coupled with papers applying grounded theory naturally offer unique empiricism within the clinical context. Engagement with [post-]positivism and interpretivism, epistemologically, and also postmodernism (methodologically) within my own PhD identifies a pluralist approach. This experience leads to accepting opposing epistemological thought, as outlined within this chapter. Whilst at a paradigmatic level, qualitative and quantitative research is considered juxtaposed (Kuhn, 1962, p.162), demonstrating two distinct paradigms, yet, it also leads to a third paradigm (Creswell and Plano Clark, 2007). Creswell and Plano Clark (2007) identified three considerations when dealing with alternate or conflicting worldviews or paradigms in mixed method research. First, pragmatism, which is considered important as it allows a researcher to focus on his/her research question, regardless of the method or philosophical worldview that underlies the method (ibid). Second, acceptance that different paradigms give rise to contradictory ideas and contested arguments (ibid) and third, it should not recognize that mixed methods are strictly a method, thus allowing researchers to employ any number of philosophical foundations for its justification and use (ibid). These assertions are helpful for a number of reasons when it comes to researching radiography. Two particular issues stand out. First, the assessment by Creswell and Plano Clark (2007) suggests that researchers need not conform or be constrained by a particular research philosophy, especially if they have a particular goal or topic of interest. For instance, you may decide to undertake an X-ray experiment for a dissertation project, but it does not mean you are a positivist, and will always be a positivist! I often hear academics dismissing or rejecting one form of philosophy, against another. As student radiographers or prospective researchers, it is important to broaden our philosophical perspectives, remain open whilst mindful that other approaches, which contribute and support, not allowing it to confine or restrict a projects intentions. Second, if undertaking postgraduate research (in particular a PhD), you will be confronted with ensuring you 'have a stance' or 'a lens'. Looking back, however, my biggest challenge was the requirement to 'pick' a philosophical lens, either at the outset or throughout my research. On reflection, this was not necessarily a failure of philosophical understanding or reasoning, but one of philosophical curiosity, which has now added value elsewhere (Hayre and Blackman, 2020; Hayre et al., 2021).

The practice of pragmatism may be exciting for mixed method researchers as it strives to bridge the gap between objectivism and subjectivism. It enables researchers to use theories, inductive reasoning, coupled with hypothetical-deductive approaches to support individualistic roles and goals at the paradigmatic level and strategically, methodologically in order to answer research questions (Creswell and Plano Clark, 2007). For a pragmatist, (s)he may need to identify a research problem in the clinical setting, which seeks to be rectified via practice solutions to inform policy and/or practice. For example, if a researcher has a specific goal that requires mixed methods then it could be accepted that a pragmatist approach can satisfy practical outcomes. It is important to note, however, that not all pragmatists will conform to alternate methods, nor does it suggest that all mixed method researchers use pragmatism (as in my experience) (ibid). For this aspect of the book it is accepted that pragmatism can pave the way for applying innovative and multi-method approaches whilst facilitating philosophical underpinnings to practical solutions, especially in the field of diagnostic radiography, which offers different forms of reasoning.

2.6 PHILOSOPHY FOR RADIOGRAPHIC RESEARCHERS?

For researchers in radiography seeking to perform qualitative or quantitative approaches, their philosophical lens may differ depending on their chosen methodology and/or methods. From experience, performing an ethnographic study may generally utilise social constructionism and interpretivism, as identified in other ethnographic works in radiography (Larsson et al., 2007; Strudwick, 2015; Nightingale et al., 2016). Yet, my decision to incorporate X-ray experiments as part of an ethnographic approach, at the time, perhaps appeared a little risky in light of some former use. At first glance, it could be assumed the abovementioned remained mixed, thus the requirement for a mixed method philosophy, perhaps pragmatism? However, the concern of accepting pragmatism was ultimately grounded on the role of a radiographer, whereby similarities as an ethnographer were noted. After careful consideration, the role of the ethnographer and radiographer share similar meanings and to ignore these would have ignored the inherent virtues, later termed 'ethno-radiographer' within postmodern ethnography (Hayre, 2016a). The importance of failing to recognize ethnography within radiographic practice offered a potential neglect of one role over another.

Since appreciating its interconnectedness, this has been expressed and translated elsewhere (Hayre and Blackman, 2020). In short, for radiography researchers, there are a number of opportunities whereby positivist, critical realist, interpretivist and postmodernist philosophies are incorporated into our everyday work. For example, as radiographers, we utilize ionizing radiation (positivism), interpret radiographs, leading to differences in opinion (critical realism), observe, monitor, interact and care with our patients (interpretivism), whilst potentially remaining suppressed by means of language and ideological radiographic doctrine (postmodernism). The views expressed here are suggesting that radiographers (along with other health professionals) remain involved in a range of ontologies and epistemologies. It is accepted that stronger philosophical traditions will remain, which are deep rooted in a particular discourse or culture of a discipline. Yet, if we accept equity amongst these philosophical schools of thought, we can acknowledge the utilitarian approaches of each.

For any given study seeking to examine new insight it will require philosophical thinking that paves the way for empirical and methodological utility in the diagnostic radiography profession and may also facilitate the development of prospective researchers now and in the future.

2.7   CHAPTER SUMMARY

This chapter began by introducing research philosophy, coupled with pertinent concepts, such as ontology and epistemology. Objective and subjective descriptors were offered in accordance with differing philosophies. A central outcome in this chapter has not been to simply regurgitate descriptors of positivism, critical realism, interpretivism and postmodernism, but to interlink these philosophies with experiences and identify alternate ways of thinking. What is affirmed is the potential for researchers to extend beyond a single philosophical norm and accept the utility of perhaps unconventional philosophies, such as postmodernism. This chapter has introduced not only the commonly regarded philosophies, but also challenges the status quo, which may encourage students to think about their philosophical journey in research. Through critical appreciation of our own ontological and epistemological assumptions and how this may differ in the profession such as diagnostic radiography, whereby we broaden our knowledge base and atypical discourses, which have remained generally accepted.

KEY TERMS

Axiology: is the philosophical study of value and can be considered a collective term for both ethics and aesthetics.

Contemporary: is associated with belonging to or occurring in the present. It can also be linked to living or occurring at the same time.

Critical realism: a branch of philosophy that distinguishes between what is deemed the 'real' world and what can be known in the 'observable' world.

Discourse: is a form of written or spoken form of debate and thus can be associated with a particular writing style which is, say, authoritative about a certain topic or phenomena.

Epistemology: is regarded as the theory of knowledge and thus how knowledge can be derived and understood. This is intrinsically linked to the methods, internal and external validity, and how it can inform an evidence base, such as radiography.

Foundationalism: is a philosophical theory of knowledge that rests upon justified beliefs or some other foundational elements in order for conclusions to be inferred.

Generalizations: is typically associated with quantitative methods and is an overarching statement that seeks to provide general statements or concepts which have been inferred.

Hypothetical-deduction: is a form of reasoning that involves starting with a general theory of all potential factors, which may then impact an outcome of an X-ray experiment. It is here, whereby deductions can be made from the hypothesis to predict outcomes from the experiment.

Interpretivist: is a branch of epistemology that assumes the potential of multiple realities via the creation of knowledge. This branch of reasoning, then, does not seek to provide generalizations, but uncover novel and deep-rooted feelings and beliefs towards a certain subject.

Logical positivism: a form of positivism that considers that only meaningful philosophical problems are those which can be solved by logical analysis.

Metaphysical: related to metaphysics, which is a branch of philosophy that deals with the first principles of things and involves conceptual modes such as being, knowing, identify, time and space.

Narrative: a narrative is a spoken or written account of connected events, i.e., a particular story. It is often associated with qualitative research and the 'narrative' surrounding an informants views or attitudes, but it can also be linked to other works.

Objectivist: is a view or tendency to emphasize what is external to or independent of the mind. Philosophically, it holds the belief that certain things, especially moral truths exist independently of human knowledge or perception of them.

Ontology: is a branch of metaphysics, which concerns and explores the nature of our reality. It, therefore, holds a set of concepts and categories within a particular subject area, or discipline, whilst showing relations between them.

Pluralist: a pluralist lens assumes that diversity is beneficial and that knowledge generation can be built from varying cultural groups with a society. This can include religious groups, professionals and ethnic minorities.

Positivism: is a form of philosophy that recognizes only what can be scientifically verified or capable of logical or mathematical proof, thus based on laws of generalization.

Post-positivism: is a branch of epistemological thought that critiques positivism whereby post-positivists argue that theories, hypotheses, background knowledge and values can all influence what is 'scientifically observed'. In short, the search for objectivity is maintained, but with potential for bias.

Postmodernism: can be seen as a reaction against the ideas and values of modernism. It can be affiliated with scepticism, irony and philosophical critiques of the concepts of universal truths and our objective reality.

Pragmatist: or pragmatism is generally recognized as a guide and answer to help practical application, rather than ideals. It can be drawn from alternate theories and discourses in order to meet an aim or objective of an intended study.

Realism: is a stance which considers phenomena representing people or thing accurately and remaining true to life.

Social constructionism: is regarded as the theory of knowledge that is based on shared assumptions, the value of multidimensional views in reality.

Subjectivism: is concerned that knowledge is merely subjective and that there is no external or objective truth, which is waiting to be measured or observed.

Theological: is the systematic study of the nature of the divine and thus broadly that of religious beliefs.

Unificationist: is typically ascribed to the advocacy and adherent of unification, which can be one of the political powers, or one of the scientific enquiries.

EXERCISES AND STUDY QUESTIONS

1   If you are about to embark on a research project, consider writing a 1,000-word reflection that examines your ontology and epistemology. When critiquing this, be mindful of your axiology, system of beliefs, views and opinions of certain topics.

2   Imagine you could forget everything you once knew – it is important as a researcher (and in particular as a PhD student) to distance yourself from what you have previously come to understand or know about a particular topic. As you have now read this chapter, critically think about your philosophical development and ask yourself how knowledge can be created in line with your enquiries?

3   Remain mindful of the opportunities a PhD has to offer in terms of critically engaging with the philosophical epistemology. I urge PhD students to immerse themselves in the literature through wider reading in order to allow for a wider appreciation of alternate and perhaps underused epistemological positions – postmodernism, for instance.

REFERENCES

Benfield, S., Hewis, J., and Hayre, C.M. (2021) Investigating perceptions of 'dose creep' amongst student radiographers: A grounded theory study. *Radiography*, 27 (20), pp. 605–610.

Benton, T. and Craib, I. (2001) *Philosophy of Social Science*. Hampshire: Macmillan.

British Institute of Radiology (2020) Guidance on using shielding on patients for diagnostic radiology applications. A joint report of the British Institute of Radiology (BIR), Institute of Physics and Engineering in Medicine (IPEM), Public Health England (PHE), Royal

College of Radiologists (RCR), Society and College of Radiographers (SCoR) and the Society for Radiological Protection (SRP). [Online] Accessible at: www.bir.org.uk/media/414334/final_patient_shielding_guidance.pdf

Couvalis, G. (1999) *The Philosophy of Science – Science and Objectivity*. SAGE: London.

Creswell, J.W. and Plano Clark, V.L. (2007) *Designing and Conducting Mixed Methods Research*. 3rd Edn. London: Sage.

Denzin, N. (1997) *Interpretive Ethnography*. London: Sage.

DiFrisco, J. (2019). Interdisciplinarity, epistemic pluralism, and unificationism. *Studies in History and Philosophy of Science Part C: Studies in History and Philosophy of Biological and Biomedical Sciences*, 74, pp. 40–44.

Haigh, F., Kemp, L., Bazeley, P., and Haigh, N. (2019) Developing a critical realist informed framework to explain how the human rights and social determinants of health relationships work. *BMC Public Health*, 19 (1571), pp. 1–12.

Hayre, C.M. (2016a) *Radiography observed: An ethnographic study exploring contemporary radiographic practice*. Ph.D. Thesis. Canterbury Christ Church University. Faculty of Health and Wellbeing.

Hayre, C.M. (2016b) 'Cranking up', 'whacking up' and 'bumping up': X-ray exposures in contemporary radiographic practice. *Radiography*, 22 (2), pp. 194–198.

Hayre, C.M. Blackman, S., Hackett, P.M.W., Muller, D., and Sim, J. (In press). Ethnography and medicine: The utility of positivist methods in ethnographic research. *Anthropology and Medicine*.

Hayre, C.M. and Blackman, S. (2020) Ethnographic mosaic approach for health and rehabilitation practitioners: an ethno-radiographic perspective. *Disability and Rehabilitation*, pp. 1–4.

Hayre, C.M., Jeffery, C., and Bungay, H. (2020) Do lead-rubber aprons always limit ionising radiation to radiosensitive organs? *Radiography*, 26 (4), pp. e264–e269.

Hayre, C.M., Blackman, S. Carlton, K., and Eyden, A. (2019) The use of cropping and digital side markers (DSM) in digital radiography. *Journal of Medical Imaging and Radiation Sciences*, 50 (2), pp. 234–242.

Hayre, C.M., Blackman, S., Hackett, P.M.W., Muller, D., and Sim, J. (In press) Ethnography and Medicine: The utility of positivist methods in ethnographic research. *Anthropology and Medicine*. https://doi.org/10.1080/13648470.2021.1893657

Holliday, A. (2016) *Doing and Writing Qualitative Research*. 3rd Edn. London: Sage.

Kilduff, M. and Mehra, A, (1997) Postmodernism and Organizational Research. *The Academy of Management Review*, 22 (2), pp. 453–481.

Kuhn, T.S. (1962) *The Structure of Scientific Revolutions*, Chicago: The University of Chicago Press.

Larsson, W., Aspelin, P., Bergquist M., Hillergard K., Jacobsson, B., Lindskold L. et al. (2007) The effects of PACs on radiographer's work practice. *Radiography*, 13 (3), pp. 235–240.

Loder, E. (2016) Qualitative research and the BMJ. *BMJ*, 352, p. i641.

Marsh, D. and Furlong, P. (2002) A Skin, Not a Sweater: Ontology and Epistemology in Political Science. In D. Marsh and G. Stoker (eds.), Theory and Methods in Political Science. 2nd Edn. Basingstoke: Palgrave, pp. 17–41.

Nightingale, J.M., Murphy, F., Eaton, C., and Borgen R. (2016) A qualitative analysis of staff-client interactions within a breast cancer assessment clinic. *Radiography*, 23 (1), pp. 38–47.

Pole, C. and Morrison M. (2003) *Ethnography for Education*. Berkshire: Open University Press.

Saks, M. and Allsop, J. (2010) *Researching Health, Qualitative, Quantitative and Mixed Methods*. London: SAGE.

Sheppard, M. (2007) *Appraising and Using Social Research in the Human Services – An introduction for Social Work and Health Professionals*. London: Kinsley.

Sherman, R.R. and Webb, R.B. (1988) *Qualitative Research in Education: A Focus and Method*. London: The Falmer Press.

Strudwick, R.M. (2015) Labelling patients. *Radiography,* 22 (1), pp. 50–55.

Weber, M. (1946) *Science as a Vocation*. In C.W. Mills (ed.). New York: The Free Press, pp. 129–156.

3 Research Essentials in Diagnostic Radiography

Christopher M. Hayre

3.1 INTRODUCTION

This chapter begins by focusing on contextualizing and conceptualizing the research problem. One of the major challenges upon reflecting on research supervision (especially at undergraduate level) is the development and refinement of research questions. It is important to highlight here that whilst this chapter seems to provide a logical answer, in reality, this is rarely the case. Students should be consciously reflexive when reading and learning about research essentials. Discussions concerning 'reflexivity' are provided at greater depth in chapters 9 and 11 and whilst specifically focus on methodology and education, I do not wish to suggest that reflexivity occurs at certain moments. Further, whilst it is important to contextualize a problem, this chapter also examines how we evaluate the literature, coupled with discerning 'the [research] problem', later refining our research questions. Lastly, although this remains the early stages of the research process, preliminary terms such as analysing, mapping and drawing conclusions remain pertinent here.

This chapter also seeks to cement the notion that research is an ongoing process that requires moving from theory to practicalities, and back by considering what is practical and how this will develop theory or lead to new knowledge. For clarity, what may be considered as a research topic now, may differ in 3–6 months and will most likely differ upon completion (Richey and Klein, 2005). This is not uncommon, thus central to not be deterred and welcome change along the way. What is important, is our ability to recognize and acknowledge steps to students, whether simply putting pen to paper, and then revising or revisiting if/when appropriate.

3.2 CONCEPTUALIZING AND CONTEXTUALIZING THE RESEARCH PROBLEM

First, neither you nor your supervisor has a crystal ball determining your research question. It is also impossible to ascertain the impact or outcome of any intended study. By conceptualizing and contextualizing your initial problem, however, we are able to develop and shape some early ideas. Often, students will have a particular theme or area of radiographic practice they wish to explore. Importantly, our concepts

DOI: 10.1201/9780367559311-3

may change over time. Speaking from experience, initial PhD interests were driven following the completion of an honours project examining scattered ionizing radiation, a quantitative and 'scientific approach'. Initial intentions as part of the PhD were to perform a number of X-ray experiments and quantify dose optimising strategies to radiosensitive organs (as previously experienced). However, upon embarking onto the PhD Studentship programme, and upon engagement with research development programmes, coincided with pivotal assistance from supervisors, my initial intentions of conducting quantitative research remained juxtaposed with the need (and gap) in literature. In short, we needed to ensure a significant level of originality. The initial intention and suggestion of a scientific-led enquiry, whilst still important, failed to offer the originality anticipated for PhD study. Upon further enquiry, this led to additional reading followed by subsequent research in the social sciences, rather than experimentally optimizing ionizing radiation and image quality. Whilst the experimental topic sparked my initial interest, the notion of moving towards a mixed methodology (at the time) was new, but also opportunistic. This enabled me to read around topics such as ethnography, phenomenology and grounded theory (detailed in chapter 8). These approaches resulted in alternate perspectives within the evidence concerning other research methodologies and methods, which at the time, offered far greater originality. Here is a learning point. This experience demonstrates that previously held concepts may require change and that as researchers we should not be deterred or disheartened if our original concepts are altered or dismissed. Looking back, the initial line of quantitative enquiry was superseded by a mixed method rationale by means of discussion with academic peers and supervisors and upon scoping the literature. Whilst perhaps unsettling at first, it paved the way for a more informed and original study.

Upon embarking onto any research activity, it is important we are able to defend our work. Looking back on my own journey, I recollect the ability to not only develop and refine a research topic, but also defend it, either with peers, research supervisors and/or formal confirmation meetings. As a research supervisor, I remind students that devising a research idea is more than simply thinking (and producing) a large list of 'things' waiting to be discovered. Instead, I ask researchers their interests, which helps ascertain what is important to them. This helps, not only with developing the methodology, but also create realistic and achievable goals. Often, there may be the temptation to identify a grandeur or large-scale plan, which is often outside the scope of any academic award. This is fine, for now. What remains important is that students continue to conceptualize and contextualize their projects by engaging in dialogue and discourse with peers and their supervisory team. It is here where support and guidance focuses on emerging concepts and begins to contextualize the problem at hand (Stone, 2002). In addition, it provides an opportunity to 'refine you' whereby supervisors redirect or simplify ideas and provide guidance on both practical (methodological) and realistic (empirical) advice on your overarching project.

As understood in chapter 2, our research ideas and focus can often be linked to our axiology, which defines our research choices and quest for knowledge in a particular domain. The skill, then, is translating these deep-rooted ideas into a tangible project, but also uncovering how the idea seeks originality. At first, it is not uncommon to maintain a broad perspective, which is either driven by some personal need for change or exploration, for instance. One key feature, at this stage of the research process, is what can be termed 'peeling away self' via an inherent requirement to critically distance oneself from our deep-rooted ideas and factor in empirical and methodological evidence (Miles et al., 2015). This does not happen in a vacuum, nor in a linear fashion (although we may like to think it does), thus acceptance to a non-linear model recognizes that upon seeking to both conceptualize and contextualize a research problem, the practice of moving back and forth is central (Aspers and Corte, 2019). From experience and in conversations with students, it is important to be open to change and remain critical of previous assumptions held within a given subject. This may require redirection of ideas and thoughts in order to succeed. In short, it is important to engage in a research process that critically explores the examination of self, as well as the research topic. This can help deliver good concepts by critically questioning and reflecting about a given topic. Reflecting back on my own studies as an undergraduate radiography student, I recognized that patients undergoing lateral radiographic examinations of the elbow would potentially be receiving scattered ionizing radiation to radiosensitive organs. This observation led to the reasoning and examination of scattered ionizing radiation to radiosensitive organs, whilst seeking to mitigate potential risk. In short, my research problem was merely a conjecture and based on observed practices as a student radiographer. After careful examination, this was later deemed to be originally important whereby upon examining the literature, few studies had explored this experimentally. This later led to the development of two journal publications that recognized the potential for both the rise and limitation of ionizing radiation to radiosensitive organs (Hayre et al., 2018; Hayre, Jeffery and Bungay, 2020).

In order to 'come up' with an idea, coincided with critically situating it within everyday practice, it is recommended that students recollect observations in practice and think about the potential impact it may have if explored within the research space. Upon thinking about a particular problem, try to think why it is important. For instance, in the example above, my inductive thoughts of scattered ionizing radiation began by thinking about the rationale of undertaking such an experiment in the first instance. For example, being reminded of the radiobiological risks, underpinned by the linear nonthreshold (LNT) dose-response model, affirming that all ionizing radiation (however small) has the potential to induce some malignant change, I began to reflect on those radiosensitive organs in close proximity to the primary beam, notably breast, thyroid and eye lens. This type of self-led enquiry reinforced the rationale for this project and supported the rationale and practical undertaking at the time. Here, it is evident that my initial idea was merely embryonic. Central, however, was later utilizing research supervisors to assist with methodological design and perform the experiment. Looking back on these experiences as both a student and as a PhD supervisor, I reflect on the former remaining paramount in my work.

Finally, whether at the early or late stages of conceptualizing and contextualizing your idea, hold onto it, but, be mindful to critique it theoretically, philosophically and methodologically. Research is interwoven philosophically and methodologically, as we will come to appreciate in chapters 5–10. This will remain pivotal upon seeking originality of an intended study whereby conjuring up an idea is important. A disconnect may also arise during the early stages in relation to 'knowing little'; but as progression is made with increased knowledge and understanding, it will be you, the researcher, that understands the topic and surrounding evidence at much greater depth.

3.3   EVALUATE EXISTING LITERATURE

Clearly, a critical research step in developing your idea or trying to 'get a feel' if your idea is unique requires examination of the literature. Literature not only helps build your knowledge base, but tells us what's out there and more importantly, what's not out there. For a good guide that underscores the common strategies, coincided with types or searches and Boolean operators, readers are encouraged to examine the article by Grewal, Kataria and Dhawan (2016). These virtues are commonplace and thus any forthcoming commentary should be supported with methodologically systematic approaches (ibid).

To begin, I am often faced with the same question from students: 'where do I start?' This is an important question and whilst perhaps wise to start with a large literature search using appropriate Boolean terms and keywords, an additional strategy may also help. By simply beginning with recently published literature in relation to a respective topic and/or area(s) of interest, it can help quickly discern originality of an idea. My reasoning for exploring this is twofold. First, recent articles provide us with contemporary insight of researchers within the discipline. Here you can immerse yourself in the authors work and familiarize yourself with their empirical findings and themes, which may closely resemble your own. Second, papers of this nature not only represent important work related to your field or specialism of interest, but also serve as a tool for highlighting areas of empirical opportunity, which may often be termed 'recommendations' within the paper itself. Here, you may be able to cast methodological assumptions on prospective ideas and/or highlight specific areas of radiographic practice currently underexplored. Further, limitations depicted in articles of interest may identify current weaknesses or gaps in the paper itself, which again, paves a way for additional work to be undertaken – the niche, for example. This is an important critique in papers whereby areas of 'research opportunity' exist for students. In short, several journal articles can provide prospective students with critical insight of issues, which are supported with undertaking systematic literature review approaches. By recognizing this, in particular in the early stages of evaluating the literature, it can help discuss/dismiss obvious areas of interest with peers and supervisors of your chosen topic.

In terms of deciding 'what literature to examine', it is important to highlight some core features in the evidence. For instance, secondary literature involves publications that interpret, analyses and evaluate evidence from primary sources. For instance, this book is regarded as secondary literature, providing an interpretive, analytical and evaluative prose of two researchers within diagnostic radiography. Clearly, our accounts are interpretive and thus based on experiences of handling, managing and publishing primary data. Other secondary sources can take the form of journal articles and books. The latter can be edited or monographic and whilst this authored book underwent a review process with a publisher prior to being commissioned, it is regarded as a secondary source. The former, however, is considered our gold standard within the discipline, whereby peer-reviewed articles are deemed high quality in relation to the peer-review process. A peer-reviewed journal article undergoes a rigorous academic process by which manuscripts (the article prior and during submission phase) can either be accepted or rejected. For instance, when crafting a manuscript, authors will send the manuscript to a respective journal. Here, Editors will oversee the manuscript and begin by discerning its applicability by examining content for the journal's readership. If the Editor considers the manuscript to have methodological or empirical significance, the Editor will send the manuscript for peer review. Invited reviewers are sought within their respective radiographic areas to perform a critique of the manuscript. Reviewers provide their feedback on the quality and focus on its methodology and empirical utility. For authors, this may lead to revision or rejection depending on its overall quality.

By understanding this process, it provides us with an appreciation of the academic rigor of published works. In addition, it emphasizes the significance of peer-reviewed articles within the radiographic literature for student radiographers (and indeed academics) entering the research world and also paramount for students seeking to establish a knowledge base, say, in another topics. Primary literature, on the other hand, is considered data that is presented in its raw form. It will have stemmed from a particular source, such as an X-ray experiment, a semi-structured interview or personal diary. When engaged in the empirical phase of the research process, it is here where you are exposed to primary data whereby interpretation, analysis and evaluation constitutes it being a secondary source.

In order to evaluate existing knowledge, it means performing a number of tasks. There are three stages which are discussed here. First, when writing either a proposal or thinking of a potential topic, it is important to imagine yourself with no knowledge. By this, it should be advocated that your evaluations of existing knowledge remain broad – do not assume that everyone knows what you know! You should initially position your topic in what we term 'broad knowledge' (Snyder, 2019). In this section, it is important to introduce the area of interest, even if it means identifying information that is widely known by your supervisors, or you. Students should evaluate the literature and situate themselves initially, but it is also important to imagine that you are writing for an audience who knows nothing about your topic. From experience, students often feel that when writing and evaluating existing knowledge for the first time, there is a possibility of focusing solely on the technical components of the literature. Importantly, however, our first stage, 'broad knowledge' should 'set the scene' and keep things simple by introducing the field, whether general radiography, computed tomography and/or ultrasound. We must also accept at this point that the reader, i.e., your supervisor, may know this 'knowledge' very well, but this should not deter you from situating your project in this space.

Second, whilst it is important to keep things broad in the initial phases, you may now wish to 'focus' and 'narrow down' your field of interest. Here, repetition should be avoided, coincided with the recommendation that when evaluating the literature, the student should begin to focus on aspects of radiography that may no longer be well known to a lay member or even a member of your supervisory team (ibid). This section, then, delves into the technical components, i.e., those relating to an imaging modality for instance, or delving into critical theory concerning patient care. In this section, students should now begin to introduce technical finesse of a given topic whereby known concepts, terms and phrases are introduced. At this point, it demonstrates that you (the author) are in a position that demonstrates sound knowledge and understanding on the given topic.

Third, upon evaluating the existing knowledge base, it will now require a finer focus. Whereas the previous two stages require both broad and technical acumen in order to position your study within the existing literature; the final section is the gap analysis (Torraco, 2005). At this critical stage, the prose moves beyond what we currently know and should now inform the reader where the gap in literature lies – the originality. Here, a clear rationale for the research is identified, i.e., the gap, the void which needs to be filled. By ending with a gap analysis, it identifies not only the search for originality, but also delineates and uncovers the need for the research to commence. Figure 3.1 demonstrates this focus and the three steps involved. It is important to highlight that the bottom of the inverted triangle is not complete and deliberately designed in order to capture and remind us that whilst you may be certain a gap exists, it does not mean that evaluation should stop. As you progress and continue to read around important topics, you will be continually cementing your gap analysis with ongoing reading and research. At this stage, it may be months or years later until it is disseminated as a journal article. Thus, within this time, you will need to have ensured to have captured other supporting literature that emerges, which will help further reinforce or minimally redefine your gap analysis. This supports the rationale for the arrow depicted in the figure in order to remain mindful of new

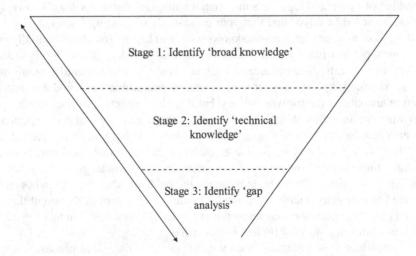

FIGURE 3.1 Approach for evaluating existing knowledge.

knowledge, which will bolster broad, technical and original assertions of the intended research. At this point, the researcher is well-positioned and has not only developed a sound knowledge base, but strategically situated the idea within the current body of knowledge – the paradigm. Whilst undergoing this process, we need to act with this information, and it is here where you can begin to write your purpose, aim and objectives and/or research questions, which are now considered.

3.4   THE 'PROBLEM' OR 'OPPORTUNITY' AND RESEARCH QUESTIONS

As progression is made, it is important to identify the 'research problem'. Considering it as a 'problem' is often the key driver for moving or engaging in research in the first place (Baumeister and Leary, 1997). But, there may be an apparent danger here. For instance, thinking there is a 'problem' concerning an aspect of radiographic practice does not always mean it is 'research problem'. For instance, to say that radiographers do not understand how to optimize computed tomography examinations, whilst problematic, in the general sense, it fails to contextualize your intended study. In short, the concept of the 'problem' may still be hard to visualize. In response, it may be best to propose the 'research problem' as a 'research opportunity'. What remains paramount is our ability to not only identify an issue, but to also 'sell it'. If a suitable research opportunity has been identified, it is critical that research questions are developed in order to help answer this opportunity. Research questions are commonly used in qualitative research, but can also be used in quantitative studies. The latter, however, is typically affiliated with a supporting [null] hypothesis. This can be found in recent works by the author in his X-ray experimental papers (Hayre et al., 2018; Hayre, Jeffery and Bungay, 2020).

Upon further reading, analysing and evaluation, the researcher becomes naturally informed by existing literature around the topic. This may sound straightforward, but in reality, it can prove difficult. If a problem or opportunity has been uncovered, coincided with supportive research questions seeking to answer the problem, it is important it contains methodological hints or insights. In short, the research questions should now begin to show some 'how to' elements when considering any undertaking of a research approach. Knowing what your problem is via immersion and, then, emersion via the evidence is clearly apparent, but how you answer this will begin to move into the realms of research methodology. For some researchers, recognition of research questions, aims and objectives may even position itself within the methodology. Yet, from experience, it is often positioned outside the methodology in order to 'set up' and position the aforementioned methodological approach, the methodological section will remain a separate section of researchers, but has importantly been 'developed' from the literature, or lack of.

3.5   ANALYSING, MAPPING AND DRAWING CONCLUSIONS

By reading the above subheading you may be thinking why 'analysing' and 'conclusions' are mentioned early in this book, especially as there has been limited discussion on methodological strategies or collection of empirical data. Here, this

40   Research Essentials in Radiography

terminology is used within a context to help to 'connect' early ideas, existing literature, research problem(s) and proposed solution(s) [research questions]. Without knowing, we are simply making assertions throughout the research process. For example, whilst our project report or thesis will be demonstrating key literature and research approaches, we are, however, as researchers continuously analytical, by refining ideas, whilst mapping thoughts and conclusions at a practical level. One obvious example of this approach is the analytical process by which qualitative researchers engage. Typically, when qualitative researchers obtain empirical data, they are required to 'make sense' of the data (Bailey, 1996). They are often presented with an array of narrative, from interview transcripts and/or observational notes (Hammersley, 1998). This is not dissimilar from the early stages of analysing, mapping and concluding the plethora of secondary sources required to formulate and focus your research topic. Figure 3.2 provides an impression of the similarities inherent with an early career researcher and those experienced as a qualitative researcher.

In addition, a key feature of most qualitative research is to not only 'make sense' of the data, but also 'tell a story' (Denzin, 1997). Here, a qualitative researcher and embryonic researcher share a common interest – they are seeking to convey meaning to information obtained. For the qualitative researcher, this is the context of primary data, whereas for the researcher, it is via secondary sources. Thus, it is important for any new researcher to ensure that their academic prose holds significance by means of what can be deemed as storytelling, even at the early stages of

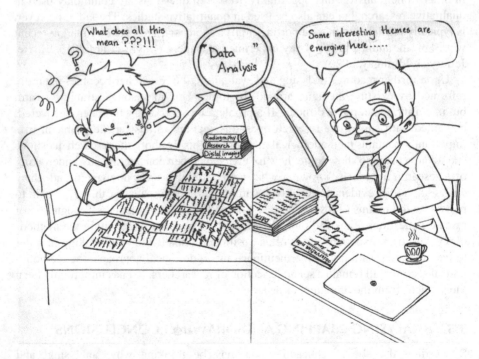

FIGURE 3.2   Similarities of 'data analysis' amongst key literature and primary qualitative data.

research. This will remain pivotal in order for your chosen topic to demonstrate meaning, purposefulness and originality in its intention to remain pertinent to the radiography profession.

When analysing and mapping previous research, you may find the need to alter its direction or purpose. An example may be where you have a particular interest to explore paediatric imaging. Yet, upon first examination, it is evident that this topic is too broad. After some further reading of the literature, you may find that research has examined the radiographer's experiences and perspective via a survey method. This tells us that perhaps there is little research that examines the patient's perspective or a radiographer's perspective from a qualitative approach, i.e., observations of paediatric imaging. Perhaps after a little more reading, you now find that research does exist which has examined the radiographers and patient's perspective via observational methods. You may, however, ask where the gap is now? Upon further investigation, you may have identified few studies exploring the caregiver's perspective during paediatric imaging. This simplistic form of refocusing has enabled us (theoretically) to determine where a potential gap may reside. This example teaches us that as we move through the literature, detours may be necessary in order to find an appropriate space [gap] which offers originality. These can be termed 'mini-conclusions' in order to seek out where the purpose is.

Further, based on the aforementioned and for, say, a research student embarking onto a PhD, students will be expected to provide enhanced contributions to the evidence base, when compared to a Master's degree. It may, then, be necessary for the student to think more broadly, methodologically, by conducting mixed methods, which not only captures caregiver's perspectives, but also seeks to record dosimetry values if/when caregivers are present in the X-ray room? Whilst this example is written on haste and without a thorough literature search, it provides an example of how ongoing analysis, [mind] mapping and drawing of conclusions will often lead to change in the researchers initial intentions in search of originality and also broadening a projects scope. It also acknowledges that it may not be necessary to make huge changes to a prospective topic or discover a grandeur topic, but about seeking out nuance differences, usually methodologically, in order to create and add substantially to your project and ultimately evidence. We also find that our search for originality can often be resolved with subtle and delicate (re)considerations from the initial scope and intentions of the research team.

In order to meet the objectives of writing and providing an evaluation of existing literature, it is recommended that new researchers analyse, map and draw conclusions continuously. For example, when finding an article that resonates with your proposed topic, it is suggested that readers offer a summary of the article, i.e., your thoughts on the content and value of the paper. This is important because it not only allows you to critically engage with the content at the time, but also enables you to integrate the text at a later date, in a thesis for instance. Upon reflecting back on what you have written, the previously paraphrased information can be readily applied into a rationale or literature review section. It is important at this stage to detail existing evidence, but also analyse, provide direction and 'hint' to the reader that a gap does exist in your related project. This will enable you to draw stronger connections with the literature and help build a robust writing and academic narrative – selling and telling your story.

The latter part of this chapter sought to link analytical, mapping and conclusive components within 'research essentials' during the early stages of research investigation. If, however, you are considering performing a quantitative experiment, this method is still suggested in accordance with the qualitative researcher. The assertion of an embryonic researcher, analogous to a qualitative researcher, is not only helpful from a practical standpoint, it also helps delineate, adjust and amend where necessary vis-à-vis, 'reflexivity in action'. Try to imagine your research proposal or protocol as a 'living document' and that whilst submitted to an ethics or confirmation panel for assessment purposes, it will always be a 'work in progress' upon considering additional research and literature. It is also important upon analysing, mapping and concluding that researchers attempt not to 'attack' literature for its lack of generalizability, for instance, or its inability to capture a particular topic in depth, but to offer a balanced prose that remains respectful to paradigmatic traditions, whilst clearly signposting the contributions of your proffered study.

3.6 CHAPTER SUMMARY

This chapter identified some early research essentials for prospective radiography researchers. The chapter began with introducing terms such as 'conceptual' and 'contextual', which will remain paramount when considering a prospective topic. It is acknowledged that this may not always be easy and may require assistance within your supervisory team. However, upon devising an idea that attempts to offer originality and remain of value, the researcher will need to explore and reevaluate existing literature. In this chapter, it is identified how researchers may wish to begin engaging in what is termed the 'broad space', which can then focus on a more 'technical' component and lastly, the gap analysis. It is strongly recommended that students do not cease evaluating the literature at this point, with recognition that ongoing reading is needed in order to reaffirm both empirical originality, coupled with methodological significance. Next, the importance of delineating the research 'problem' or 'opportunity' is helped by reflecting on the aforementioned literature search, supported with prospective solutions, notably, research questions. Lastly, a link during the early stages is made in accordance with qualitative researchers. The first author [CH] has directly experienced qualitative research, coincided with its similarities to 'starting out' in the literature. It is important, however, to highlight that whilst these 'stages' of the research process are disconnected, for now, it offers a practical guide for student radiographers seeking to make sense of the vast information currently exposed.

The thoughts and processes presented in this chapter are predominately based on previous experience with undergraduate and postgraduate research students. It is anticipated that this chapter will help overcome any confusion and natural feelings of 'feeling lost within the literature'. Yet, ideas identified here aim to provide an alternate form of considering some early stages of research development and thinking. As experienced with writing this book, our ideas not only stem from our data, but data will also influence our ideas.

KEY TERMS

Aim: is associated with having intention or intentions of achieving a desired outcome.

Analysing: seeks to examine something methodically and in meticulous detail. The overall purpose of this is to either further explain or interpret information, such as primary or secondary sources.

Conceptualizing: is regarded as the formation of a particular idea or concept of something, such as a 'research idea'.

Contextualizing: is interwoven with conceptualizing because it tends to place the idea in a relative context, such as the clinical practice context in radiography.

Empirical: is concerned with verifiable and 'trusted' research data and have usually undergone rigorous peer review in order to be accepted within an academic community.

Evaluative: is based on the critical assessment of ideas or a set of information.

Interpretive: is related to providing an interpretation of a particular set of events or information.

Mapping: is associated with the practice of examining a single aspect with one or more elements. It enables prospective researchers to compare and contrast evidence that remains important to their area of interest.

Methodological: is related to a set of methods and principles used in a particular domain or area of study.

Monographic: this relates to the word 'monograph' and whilst is affiliated with an art exhibition or gallery that showcases works by a single artist, it is also closely affiliated with single-authored books.

Objectives: is usually a set of criteria which will help achieve studies overarching aim. They can be affiliated with instruction that encompasses actions by the researcher.

Reflexive: is considered as a meaning that is directed or turned back onto itself. It can refer to individuals or particular action or process by researchers in order to provide critical insight into the actions and behaviours of self.

Research problem: is a particular area of interest selected by a researcher. It may have close associations with the researcher as they seek to provide insight into this understudied area.

Research questions: are a set of questions that seek to provide solution to a research problem. These should be devised carefully and not overcomplicated. They are also typically aligned to qualitative research, but can be used in quantitative research.

Rigor: is typically associated with intense academic quality, which has undergone extreme thought-provoking assessment.

Theoretical: is concerned with or involving theory of a particular subject rather than its practical application.

EXERCISES AND STUDY QUESTIONS

1   At the early stages of your research, it is important to write down a number of areas of research interests. This will help your research supervisor assess the applicability and practicalities of your interests depending on the academic reward in which you are working towards.

2   Upon immersion within the literature ensure you continuously reflect on your
     aim, objectives and research questions. Be mindful these will alter, which is
     fine. It will be useful to prepare this in early meetings with supervisors.
3   Ask yourself a critical question. What do you want to get out of this project?
     Once you have asked this question, ask this second question: what do you
     think you can practically achieve in this research project? When answering
     these questions be mindful of your project timeline.

REFERENCES

Aspers, P. and Corte, U. (2019) What is qualitative in qualitative research. *Qualitative Sociology.* 42, pp. 139–160.

Bailey, C.A. (1996) *A Guide to Field Research.* California: Sage.

Baumeister, R.F. and Leary M.R. (1997) Writing narrative literature reviews. *Review of General Psychology.* 1, pp. 311–320.

Denzin, N. (1997) *Interpretive Ethnography.* London: Sage.

Grewal, A., Kataria, H., and Dhawan, I. (2016) Literature search for research planning and identification of research problem. *Indian Journal of Anesthetics.* 60(9), pp. 635–639.

Hammersley, M. (1998) *Reading Ethnographic Research.* 2nd Edn. London: Wesley Longman.

Hayre, C.M. Jeffery, C., and Bungay, H. (2020) Do lead-rubber aprons always limit ionising radiation to radiosensitive organs? *Radiography.* 26(4), pp. e264–e269.

Hayre, C.M. Bungay, H., Jeffery, C., Cobb, C., and Atutornu, J. (2018) Can placing lead-rubber inferolateral to the light beam diaphragm limit ionising radiation to multiple radiosensitive organs? *Radiography.* 24(1), pp. 15–21.

Miles, M., Chapman, Y., and Francis, K. (2015) Peeling the onion: understanding others' lived experience. *Contemporary Nurse.* 50(2–3), pp. 286–295.

Richey, R.C. and Klein, J,D, (2005) Developmental research methods: Creating knowledge from instructional design and development practice. *Journal of Computing in Higher Education.* 16(2), pp. 23–38.

Snyder, H. (2019) Literature review as a research methodology: An overview and guidelines. *Journal of Business Research.* 104(1), pp.333–339.

Stone, P. (2002) Deciding upon and refining a research question. *Palliative Medicine. Issues in Research.* 16(1), pp. 265–267.

Torraco, R.J. (2005) Writing integrative literature reviews: Guidelines and examples. *Human Resource Development Review.* 4(1), pp. 356–367.

4 Ethical Considerations in Radiography Research

Christopher M. Hayre

4.1 INTRODUCTION

Research ethics remains integral in all prospective studies with the overall aim of protecting individuals. This chapter discusses ethical principles and practices based on current literature and via experience of undertaking both qualitative and quantitative research in radiography. Ethics has its roots in the ancient Greek philosophical enquiry of moral life. Ethics is about critically challenging decision making, which can open up new discussions and ways of practicing in research. This means it is not static and can evolve depending on new methodological strategies or insights. Importantly, it seeks to discern what is right from wrong (Pole and Morrison, 2003). This chapter begins by discussing the role of research ethics within the research process, which leads to a gap analysis. It is imperative that these two features are understood prior to considering ethical approval. The decision was made to discuss ethics at this stage of the book (chapter 4) because it is important to understand some core principles behind research ethics prior to considering a methodology. This may help construct your own research methodology, but researchers may prefer to engage in the methodological chapters before considering ethical principles. Naturally, one will always inform the other in terms of trying to understand the type of methodology in response to the research question(s). Other topical discussions not only identify ethical principles, but are supported with first-hand experience. In addition, this chapter sets a narrative for moving beyond pre-empirical ethical considerations and discusses how researchers remain 'ethically minded' post-empiricism, and into dissemination. This leads us to answer an important question: Does the ethical process stop?

4.2 ROLE OF RESEARCH ETHICS AND HISTORICAL CONTEXT

Ethics is concerned with moral questions and issues that arise in light of prospective research studies (Pole and Morrison, 2003). Having chaired and been a member to various ethics committees in different parts of the world, my lens is fairly broad, having been either a reviewer and overall decision-maker. A principle concern in social science research is the role human participants' play when being involved

DOI: 10.1201/9780367559311-4

in research, which can differ depending on the topic and/or local culture (Dimond, 2002). Because ethics is about examining the moral life and discerning right from wrong, researchers must accept that these 'rights and wrongs' may differ depending on the country and/or alternate cultures. Furthermore, it is imperative, as researchers, to remain mindful of alternate customs and norms thus having an inherent duty of care to our prospective participants' health and well-being. This can range from ensuring that individuals are able to self-determine, have privacy and that information concerning individuals is kept confidential (Hammersley, 1998). As we will appreciate, the role of ethics does not begin and end with the research ethics committee. It is inherent throughout the research process and recognizing this will provide a more holistic approach for an approved project.

A pertinent question that can be asked is: why do we have ethical standards? Whilst the answer is perhaps obvious, as researchers must ensure the rights and welfare of research participants are protected. In addition to this, ethical procedures are also in place to protect you, the researcher and ensure that the accuracy of scientific knowledge is continuously upheld. There are examples where research has caused much confusion and inaccuracy via the reporting of research data (Kingori and Gerrets, 2016). Obvious mistreatment of research subjects can be linked to research that has been carried out without ethical approval, or complete failure to follow approved protocols, whilst identifying absent or inadequate informed consent forms or failures to maintain appropriate confidentiality.

The ongoing rationale for research ethics and why it remains paramount is best reminded by looking back on how researchers behaved inappropriately in the past, leading to what is now regarded as unethical research. Unethical research closely resembles those practiced during the Second World War, whereby Nazi scientists performed a number of experiments on prisoners, including children, from across Europe. The concentration camps were withholding prisons during World War II are commonly referred to as 'The Holocaust'. The coerced prisions did not volunteer, nor was there any consensual responses, with many of the experiments in which individuals were exposed led to death, disfigurement and/or permanent disability (Jotkowitz, 2008). In short, these examples (of which were conducted for medical purposes) are today considered examples of medical torture.

A number of examples are well cited within the literature, including experiments on twin children; bone, muscle and nerve transplantation; head injury experiments; and freezing experiments (Weindling et al., 2016). In addition, the Tuskegee syphilis experiment during 1932–1972 is now regarded as unethical research (Mata et al., 2016). This study was conducted by the US Public Health Service, monitoring more than 600 low-income black American males (400 of whom were infected with syphilis for 40 years). Whilst free medical examinations were given, individuals were not treated or told about the disease, despite a proven cure, penicillin, readily available at the time (ibid). Many of the individuals during this study died of syphilis. The study was finally stopped in 1973 by the US Department of Health, Education and Welfare because its existence became public knowledge. In 1997, the US President, Bill Clinton issued a formal apology.

There are now codes of ethical practice that all researchers should abide. First is the 1947 Nuremberg Code, created following the Nuremberg trials at the end of the Second World War, identifying the importance of voluntary consent. It contains 10 ethical principles (World Health Organization, 2021) which remain central for guiding researchers ensuring that efforts are made to limit harm to participants. In addition, the 1964 Declaration of Helsinki remains endorsed by the World Medical Association (WMA) offering statements of ethical principles for medical research involving human subjects (WMA, 2021). Whilst we appreciate that research at an early career level is unlikely to involve medical research *per se*, it is important to be guided by these ethical principles and also mindful of implications upon research with participants.

4.3 PRINCIPLES PROTECTING HUMAN PARTICIPANTS

As a student radiographer and/or practicing radiographer, we have an inherent need to ensure we protect those around us. Remember, good and well-designed studies advance the evidence base, whereas poorly conducted studies violate the principle of justice and become a wasted resource for the extension of academic knowledge (Petre and Rugg, 2004). Arguably, then, our principle of protecting patients as we [you] become healthcare professionals will not only resonate, but remains applicable to the research context. For instance, if deciding to embark into research which is not anthropomorphic, which requires human participation, we must consider both moral and ethical implications of these individuals. The four main areas recognized here (and elsewhere) are beneficence, non-maleficence, respect for persons (autonomy) and justice.

Beneficence: considers balancing benefits of treatment against the risks and costs. In our everyday radiographic practice, this is correlated with the practice of justification, whereby radiographers expose a patient to ionizing radiation *if* the radiological exposure can benefit the patient in some way – diagnosis. Similarly, in research, researchers should only be involving participants if their involvement will benefit the intended aim and research question(s) of the study. This Hippocratic principle of 'be of benefit, do not harm' seeks to serve and promote the welfare of individuals in society; however, it can often be challenging when designing research questions, in particular, qualitative studies (Ashcroft et al., 2007). For example, the exploratory nature of qualitative research offers unpredictability, thus by ensuring beneficence requires an on-going critique and reflexive process built on published works and engagements with ethics committees. These, to some degree help reaffirm the intention of beneficence to the individuals it involves.

Non-maleficence: focuses on the avoidance of harm and any subsequent risks to a participant (Saks and Allsop, 2010). Non-maleficence requires a level of sensitivity from the researcher about what constitutes 'harm' by ensuring not only prevention, but limitation. It should consider possible actions and how the researcher seeks to balance risks with proportionate benefits. In short, as healthcare professionals, we do not intend to 'harm' our patients and whilst there is some acceptance that hazards exist for certain procedures by means of stochastic effects, we should not deliberately overexpose patients or deliberately perform more radiographs than necessary, this is unethical practice. When examining this in the research context, then, it may involve asking sensitive questions that are controversial, inappropriate and/or perhaps considered unethical. We should remain mindful as researchers that our positionality (discussed more in chapter 9) may cause unintentional discomfort to participants (Hayre and Hackett, 2020). Whilst undeliberate, it is critical to reflect on our verbal and non-verbal cues and those reactions of participants in order to balance asking pertinent and original questions, with ethical and moral virtues in place.

Respect for persons (autonomy): this principle is generally focused on accepting and respecting the decision-making of individuals. Typically, when conducting research on research participants, it is important to recognize an individual's autonomous decision-making. This involves an appreciation that individuals make reasoned and informed choices. Whilst a heightened discussion point, reflecting on my own radiographic practice whereby patients refuse to undergo an X-ray examination can be either accepted or rejected, depending on the patients' capacity to decide. Clearly, in research, and research we are most likely to be involved in, the former is commonplace. In situations where participants generally have the capacity to reason and consent into a research study, we must accept the participant's decision to enter the study or not.

Justice: the notion of justice can be linked to radiography research. For instance, if a group of participants have consented to take part in a study, it is essential for synonymous treatment. This is important when it comes to ensuring that participants are fully informed about the research process, via a participant information sheet (PIS), for instance. A PIS is a central piece of accompanying documentation that asks 'lay questions', with little jargon and descriptive [lay] answers. Here, participants are exposed to questions that details the purpose of the study, involvement required and time period. Whilst patients may be invited to take part in prospective studies, it is also important their input is heard. For instance, reflecting upon the moderation of two focus groups of people with dementia, seeking encouragement from all participants was key, enabling the expression of ideas and experiences. Another example relates to the conducting of surveys of undergraduate radiography students whereby all members of a cohort are heard in order to capture a diverse set of perspectives.

The abovementioned is generally recognized within the literature (Ashcroft et al., 2007). The discussion will now identify four further items; disclosure, confidentiality, participation and consent.

4.3.1 Disclosure

When considering disclosure, some interesting discussions emerge. Ideas surrounding disclosure link to whether participants are ever fully aware of a researcher's intentions? Whilst some of this narrative surrounds involvement in randomized controlled trials (RCT), for instance, whereby informing participants may also impede research outcomes in placebo situations, the notion of fully disclosing the researcher's interests and goals, may also be hidden within social science research (Hayre, 2016). There is some debate that researchers 'have their own agendas' and intention in research which are never perhaps fully disclosed. Little is written about disclosure within the radiography literature but, here, it is acknowledged that researchers continuously strive to disclose information and research intentions to gatekeepers and participants throughout the research process. In my view, it is paramount that researchers seek to fully disclose what is necessary and within the ethical boundaries of the research. One clinical example resonates in our everyday practices in radiography whereby some radiographers were observed not disclosing obvious osseous fractures to patients (Hayre, 2016). This phenomenon has emerged in recent years due to the immediate reviewing of digital radiographs in the X-ray room, whereas historically, images/ films were reviewed outside the X-ray room and away from the patient's suspicion. I have observed and experienced this phenomena personally, whilst grappling with the challenges of either providing the patient or caregiver a verbal diagnosis or not. This is an important area for discussion because there is already a potential discrepancy with 'radiographic disclosure' in our everyday practices by not disclosing fractures that are perhaps obvious and arguably within the scope of a radiographers practice. This example recognizes that disclosure may not always be binary, and in some circumstances covert, yet, it is important that our actions as researchers and practitioners are performed openly and honestly in order to uphold both clinical and research practices.

4.3.2 CONFIDENTIALITY

Anonymity means to disguise or remove the identity of participants. This is important when disseminating research that is read, say, by the radiographic community. Whilst pseudonyms are important and commonly used in qualitative research in order to prevent the identification of participants individually, there are other possible identifiers that may inadvertently lead to the identification of participants or hospital sites in radiography. For instance, the geographical location, i.e., *East of England*, coupled with a radiographer's rank, i.e., *Consultant Radiographer* could be delineated by others in response to a small number of *Consultant Radiographers* in the *East of England*. This is just one example, which may not directly name or identify an individual, but indirectly allows readers to 'filter' and recognize individuals or hospital locations.

Above all, anonymization helps researchers meet data protection requirements in their respective countries, such as the Data Protection Act (2018) in the United Kingdom. This piece of legislation ensures that data should only be held for a period of time and later destroyed when it is no longer needed. One obvious practice of maintaining anonymity throughout research is by not collecting identifiable data in the first instance. Codes, or numbers, could be used in association with participants, thus immediately preventing identification with the researcher during the analytical process. Whilst useful, it may not always be practical, especially if sequential methods are utilized whereby follow-up interviews or focus groups are required with specific participants (Baily, 1996). Thus in order to ensure confidentiality, we should remain mindful of protecting individuals from 'identifiable harm'. An obvious example from experience upon examining ethical applications involves the exploration of gang crime/culture. This clearly raises ethical considerations whereby the identification of respondents has potential detriments to the health and well-being of those taking part, including the researcher(s). For radiography research, this is also important, whilst we may not closely resemble heightened risks, as identified above, we should be mindful of our confidentiality practices that protect our colleagues, patients and other individuals involved in the study. For instance, in previous radiography research, observing and interacting with radiographers over a period of 4 months led to unique and previously unaccounted data from practicing radiographers. Yet, some of the respondents' comments could have been viewed as unprofessional, inappropriate or even unethical by members of the radiographic community. Looking back, this highlighted that if confidential practices were not strictly adhered, in both the thesis write up and dissemination phase, radiographers could be made vulnerable within the workplace, if identified indirectly, and perhaps within the wider professional community. Thus, to uphold the confidentiality of participants, we remind researchers here that confidentiality should be closely affiliated with 'beneficence' – the virtue of doing no harm to participants, which falls within the form of disclosure either directly or indirectly. On the other hand, there has to be some acceptance and rationality for breaching the confidentiality of participants. For example, if upon observation, a radiographer physically assaulted a patient or acted in a way that would be deemed illegal or grossly unprofessional, it would need to be reported. These events are highly unlikely and thankfully unobserved from experience, but require acknowledgement and incident reporting. Further, although unlikely, the possibility of observing illegal or unethical behaviour should remain at the forefront in some research due to its exploratory and inductive nature, leading to unexpected results.

Looking back from experience, the use of flow charts helped signpost appropriate reporting methods if gross practices were observed. A flow chart not only helped facilitate my method of managing a potential unethical situation, but also accepted the possibility of observing and, then, acting on those practices observed in the clinical environment (Bailey, 1996). The idea of upholding confidentiality outside of serious misconduct should be carried out throughout the research process and also encouraged to encapsulate at hospital sites. An emerging area included in the research process is the use of social media and/or use of photographs or videos. Whilst appropriate approval should be collected in all cases, the latter is more complex and advised that researchers seek consent of photography or videography involving participants (regardless of whether the participants face is seen or not). Personal experiences as an editor suggests that such approval from clients or participants remains essential for researchers progressing if uploading photographic material and thus included in subsequent ethics applications, if necessary.

Lastly, from an empirical standpoint, whilst keeping participants and locations confidential is morally and ethically 'the right thing to do', it importantly leads to richer data, especially in qualitative research. Looking back, participants who know that their feelings, thoughts and attitudes will not be traced back to them will naturally offer deeper and richer responses to questions posed (Pole and Morrison, 2003). This, in turn, will lead to enhanced empirical outcomes for any intended research study.

4.3.3 PARTICIPATION

Whilst diagnostic radiography has historically focused on experimental research and remains aligned to positivism, there is a growing body of literature that continues to examine the radiography profession from a social anthropological lens. In light of this growing trend, it is ethically and morally important to consider professional and environmental factors, as well as the researcher's role. Radiographers embarking into research may find themselves faced with competing duties, obligations and/or conflicts of interests, coincided with the necessity of making choices in the field. One example, stemming from my PhD work was captured upon observing radiographers operating digital X-ray equipment. A key research question in my PhD was the examination of ionizing radiation, yet, on some occasions radiographers would fail to select the appropriate digital detector prior to irradiating the patient. As a registered healthcare professional, it was my duty, upon anticipation, to notify the radiographer of their mistake in order to prevent a patient from receiving a dose of ionizing radiation without net benefit (no image) (Hayre, 2016). On the one hand, this intervention could arguably be interpreted as having a conflicting role in light of my anthropological role in capturing the environment in its 'natural state'. Yet, on the other hand, my own ethical and moral obligations were to the patient and radiographer, as a register radiographer myself. The former, however, whilst an 'empirical loss', offered greater methodological insight and duty whereby notifying the radiographer prevented the patient from receiving an unnecessary dose of ionizing radiation. This example demonstrates how, as researchers, our overall premise can 'anticipate harm' in the field, and that whilst observed events may lead to potential harm, there is always the possibility of unintentional and human error, which should be mitigated against whenever possible (Hayre, 2016). This example demonstrates the interconnectivity between the role of the researcher in terms of knowledge inquiry, but also his/her obligations as a registered healthcare practitioner.

Other examples, which perhaps occur within an unmeasured space is the dialogue and appropriateness of gaining access, meeting gatekeepers, appropriate attire and maintaining access. These are perhaps performed within the boundaries as both a healthcare professional and as a researcher (Bailey, 1996). Whilst the two roles could be seen as separate, they remain interlinked throughout any participatory event, whereby peers, supervisors, patients, colleagues and participants are encompassed under this umbrella of ensuring sound research delivery. Further, research projects, seeking to remain 'ethically mindful' to the participants it serves, should reflect on who is participating, and why. Upon seeking to recruit participants, it is important to identify advantages and disadvantages, and the use of inclusion and exclusion criteria. Participants may find being involved in research advantageous because the phenomenon is close to them. Further, by engaging in the research process itself, participants can learn from the process and be 'impactful' in their practices and/ or personal situations. Disadvantages may reflect the contribution of time amongst participants. For instance, you may need to obtain several hours of the participants' time when interviewing or undertaking a focus group (Saks and Allsop, 2010). This may require participation outside of their day-to-day environment or require flexibility from the primary investigator in order to meet the participant's needs, meeting at 'quieter times' – Saturday mornings, for instance (Hayre, 2016). Other disadvantages considered by participants may involve the type of questioning and/ or topic on offer. The sensitive nature, for instance, of some topics may invoke either dismay or emotion, especially if it resembles a critical moment in the participants' past. What remains central is that researchers have the appropriate responses and services available to their participants if sensitive questioning or topics arise, which puts the participants in either a vulnerable or emotional state.

What remains central is the need for good relations with all participants. It is likely your participant will not have been involved as a participant before, thus our behaviour, attitude and approachability remain paramount in order to provide a positive experience for the participant (Saks and Allsop, 2010). Research involving the social sciences often involves close and ongoing communication with participants, thus building rapport, trust, and remaining reliable and accountable to ensure sound relationships (Sheppard, 2007). In my experience, there is also a natural power differential between the participant and researcher, especially within observational research whereby the primary role of an observer is to capture the practices and behaviours of radiographers. This can lead to awkward and even hostile encounters amongst some, thus respecting potential for intrusion, with necessary scenario planning to either suspend or cease research may be necessary (Hayre and Hackett, 2020).

Central in anthropological work is the need to protect those involved in the research process, thus researchers are obliged to maintain the rights, dignity, interests and privacy of those involved (either directly or indirectly) (Hammersley, 1998). Similarly, as radiographers, our patients remain the priority in our work. Thus for researchers, this is transferable to our participants whereby the rights of participants, and gatekeepers (and patients, if necessary) come first. It is argued here that diagnostic radiography is still a 'closed profession'. Is it not uncommon for radiographers to perform X-ray examinations in a locked X-ray room, based on the rationale that colleagues could enter and become exposed to ionising radiation? This private encounter, could naturally lead to radiographers feeling that their professional space is being intruded, which should be respected. In response to my observations, it is important that upon undertaking any fieldwork in medical imaging that researchers do not overpower or impede the radiographer's ability to perform examinations safely. This may not resonate with other imaging modalities, such as CT or MRI environments, whereby control rooms are separate from the imaging rooms for safety concerns. Further, whereas radiographers generally work collegially on a single examination in either CT or MRI, the practice of general radiography and ultrasound often requires one-to-one care with patients throughout the imaging process. This relationship is not only important in terms of maintaining person-centred care, but also critical for the 'researcher–radiographer–patient' relationship whereby limited space and confidential discussions are heard. Looking back, it was important to provide as much distance as possible, hence my positioning behind the protective lead screen in the X-ray room. Not only did this protect myself from scattered ionizing radiation, but allowed the practitioner–patient examination to unfold as naturally as possible. There were, however, occasions that remained problematic due to room design and small protective spaces (Hayre, 2016). This often required abandonment of observations, especially if multiple radiographers were assisting with a single examination.

Researcher participation can be exciting, but it can also be unpredictable and depends on the environment and area of imaging, room design, patient condition and participants themselves. It is important to remember that whilst you may have consented a radiographer into your study, it does not mean it grants 'automatic access'. Consent closely aligns with these situations, as we will come to appreciate.

It is neither static nor binary. It may also move beyond formal consensual processes for medical imaging whereby continuous negotiating takes place with radiographers and/or patients in our clinical setting.

4.3.4 CONSENT

Consent is an essential part of the research process. As previously acknowledged, however, the participation of covert research negates the need to collect consent from participants by ensuring the researcher remains incognito, thus preventing the researcher from 'giving away' his/her position to respondents (Petticrew et al., 2007). The focus here, however, is the need for consent within overt research; types of consent available, supported with the rationale. When seeking consent from participants, the most common approach is informed consent, which captures a participants' voluntary request to participate in research via documentation (Bailey, 1996; Saks and Allsop, 2010). Collecting informed consent is generally accepted to be a good measure of ascertaining whether a patient's right to autonomy has been protected. This is important. Autonomy is our ability to self-determine whether we 'act' according to our personal needs, hence any informed consensual process seeks to incorporate the rights of autonomous individuals and helps uphold the integrity of the participant by balancing the risks versus benefits (Pole and Morrison, 2003). This process enables a person to voluntarily confirm his or her willingness to proceed in a study, after being informed of its intention via the PIS, as outlined above. A central feature prior to gaining informed consent is recognition of the right to refuse involvement, without reprisal or detriment to professional (or personal) relationship. This raises an important issue about educators researching students in higher education settings. For instance, with colleagues in a previous project it was decided to examine radiography students' feedback in our higher education setting. Upon seeking the necessary ethical clearance to proceed, two focus groups were formed in order to collect insightful information. Prior to this, we were conscious of our professional positions for mediating the focus groups, being the student's educators, examiners and reviewers of their academic work. This may have placed the students [participants] in a potential imbalance of power (although students were asked to take part voluntarily), which could have hindered certain responses. In order to overcome this, it was decided to ask a colleague from an external institution to mediate the focus groups, with clear recognition she sought to remain unbiased, and as 'an outsider'. Whilst satisfactory at the time, supported with a voluntary acceptance amongst students, there is still potential for cohesion. Looking back, whilst recognising our potential impact as focus group mediators, there are still potentially other inherent biases that may result if academics intend to 'research' students. In order to overcome potential imbalances, prospective researchers should think critically about the recruitment process and assess if there are alternatives that either mitigate or limit power imbalances in this context.

Informed consent sheets can be devised by the researcher or may be readily preformatted within higher education institutions. Regardless of the design, the consent process should begin with the researcher(s) ensuring the form is written in a language easily understood by individuals. It must minimize the possibility of coercion or undue influence, thus any potential participants must be given an appropriate amount of time to read and decide whether to take part or not. This is an important learning point to reflect upon. From previous work, the desire to invite diagnostic radiographers was first performed by placing A4 posters within the radiography department(s) in order to forewarn participants of my arrival – these were placed in staff rooms and in the X-ray corridor (Hayre, 2016). Further, it was decided that the PIS could be electronically sent to participants via email, as radiographers may not have been accessible if visited on a set date in response to varying shift patterns. In doing so, it sought to provide greater exposure of the intended research project, prior to attending in person. This offered additional opportunities for participants to be warned and provided with enough information and time for them to think about my intentions and decide whether to take part or not.

There is another component which warrants discussion. Verbal consent. Verbal consent is rarely discussed as a conventional consensual practice in radiography research, yet, verbal consent is used on a day-to-day basis by student radiographers and also utilized elsewhere (Lawton et al., 2017). Whilst informed consent from radiographers remained essential, verbal consent was necessary in order to gain acceptance from patients during their radiographic examinations (even though my research at the time was not directly involving patients). This indirect involvement with patients used verbal consent in order to ensure patients were happy with my presence as a researcher. In order to overcome this, it was felt that the role as a research observer mimicked the role of a student radiographer (Hayre, 2016). In general, radiography students worldwide take part in observing and learning from their clinical supervisors and either observe and/or participate in radiographic examinations. In these scenarios, verbal consent is sought from the patient prior to students being allowed to either observe and/or position the medical imaging examination. If a patient verbally accepts the student's presence and role in the X-ray room, he/she natrually observes or performs the examination under direct supervision of the radiographer. On the contrary, a patient may also refuse, which would result in the student leaving the X-ray room. This is an important consideration for prospective researchers in radiography whereby verbal consent not only plays an integral role in the everyday learning and education of students clinically, but may also play a future role in prospective research. This consensual process has been recognized in the author's work (Hayre, 2016), but perhaps lays the foundation for other types of consensual processes in radiographic research, which typically relies upon informed measures.

In some scenarios, researchers may observe patients undergoing medical imaging examinations within the emergency setting. Whilst for most patients, they will remain conscious and able to consent, verbally. However, it is possible that some patients are unconscious. This may include patients with acute head injuries or those with a suspected stroke. In these situations, researchers may want to question how consent should be gained. Two aspects stand out. First, a pertinent question should be whether the researcher needs to be in the X-ray room for the examination? For example, if the research question does not directly link to unconscious patients or examinations involving acute head injuries, then, the researcher could exit the room. On the other hand, if a key feature of the research explores how unconscious patients are treated or managed within general radiography, then this will remain a critical examination. In this instance, the ability to observe the scenario whereby current guidelines by the Council for International Organisation of Medicine Sciences, World Health Organisation and Declaration of Helsinki do make exceptions to the requirement for informed consent in situations where a patient's capacity is hindered. It is important to highlight that reasonable effort should be made in order to find a legal authority to consent, perhaps a caregiver accompanying the patient, or wherever possible, obtain informed consent from the patient when the patient regains capacity.

For researchers seeking empiricism pertinent to paediatric imaging, we are also required to think laterally in terms of consensual processes. For example, whilst consent is typically associated with adults, the term 'assent' is considered best practice for children (Field and Behrman, 2004). The term 'assent' refers to verbal or written agreement to engage in a research study, which is typically applied to children aged between 8 and 18 years. It is, however, in line with the developing capacity of the child over time and been suggested that children cannot fully consent to research from a legal perspective (ibid). Assent, then, is regarded as an affirmative agreement from the child to take part and is seen as an interpersonal act of actively participating in a process, or by verbally saying either 'yes' or 'no' (Field and Behrman, 2004). Assent is more appropriate in assessing agreement with younger children, whereas older children may respond better with more formal consensual procedures. There are few studies that focus on paediatric forms of imaging in radiography, but anticipated that with correct consensual applications and wider discussion amongst practitioners and researchers, the process of recruiting and collecting data on children will only enhance our evidence-based and research practices.

4.4   POST STUDY APPROVAL AND MONITORING

It is often a proud moment for researchers following the success of an ethics application. It is also important, however, that researchers remain 'ethically minded' throughout their research study. For instance, if undertaking research whereby you are permitted to enter a clinical environment, it will offer unpredictability with perhaps events previously unbeknown from a research perspective. This unpredictability associated with exploratory studies may lead to instances whereby researchers are required to act or respond ethically and sometimes intervene, as alluded previously (Hayre, 2016). The requirement to intervene is an example of 'ethics in action', whereby the prevention of over irradiation, facilitation of patient transfers, offering advice, and/or attempting to stop patients from falling were encountered (ibid). These are 'knee jerk' reactions whereby simply not conforming or engaging at the time could have been viewed as 'unethical or immoral reasoning'. Further, without such intervention, patients would have either been exposed to unnecessary ionizing radiation, experienced delays in imaging procedures and/or perhaps suffered other injuries whilst in the radiographers care (Hayre, 2016). In short, ethical considerations and practices of the researcher do not cease upon approval from an awarding ethics committee. Instead, there is a continuation of the virtues and principles outlined in the ethics application, which are now to be applied, methodologically. Throughout the study, it is the ethical and moral duty of researchers, but perhaps more importantly for healthcare researchers, in response to professional regulatory requirements, to ensure no harm comes to patients or peers within any setting (Pole and Morrison, 2003). By simply not intervening, this would have naturally felt juxtaposed to my professional and ethical duties as a registered diagnostic radiographer.

These experiences identify that 'who we are' both professionally and personally cannot be mitigated against and whilst emphasis focuses on the prevention of 'going native', the researcher will naturally be influenced by the environment in radiographic practice. Research, then, does not seek to negate our professional or personal virtues, instead it should be used to facilitate and build relationships in the research setting (Sheppard, 2007). As a researcher and radiographer, we perhaps build on from our skills to seek out what is ethically right and wrong from our research and clinical experiences. Here, this is recognized as 'monitoring' and I urge researchers to monitor their surroundings and act in a manner that is deemed morally and ethically right, to them, in order to avoid discomfort, or potential harm or distress to those involved in the study.

4.5   DOES THE ETHICAL PROCESS STOP?

This question is important to reflect upon because as identified above, we are continuously monitoring our surroundings in the field (Dimond, 2002). However, what happens when researchers finally leave the field? Whilst some discussion concerning this is held in chapter 11, the notion of poor ethical behaviour is typically affiliated with researchers inventing or fabricating findings in order to enhance their research (Kingori and Gerrets, 2016). This, coupled with the manipulation of collected data, which is falsification, constitutes to serious scientific misconduct. Thus, when starting out on a research journey, it is imperative that we uphold principles by presenting research in a robust and precise way. From experience, data is exciting, and can often lead to 'unexpected' findings (Hayre, Jeffery and Bungay, 2020). Whilst our initial research intentions may not have been apparent, it does not mean that the rules of ethical practice are changed. On the contrary, all data performed in a rigorous way can still add to our knowledge.

It is generally accepted that upon leaving the research environment or ceasing data collection, this could be considered the end for the ethical journey. To some degree, this is valid whereby the principle purpose safeguards participants who are involved in data collection. However, ethical committees may also consider existential factors beyond the data collection process, such as dissemination of data and supporting identifiers, as previously mentioned. Moreover, whilst physical contact may have ceased with participants, researchers are still ethically obliged to maintain contact with his/her participants in examples of member checking upon data analysis (see more in chapter 10). This is also necessary in relation to ensuring that both data and participants are accessible for robust audit trails, if required. A consideration beyond the data collection phase is dissemination. First, the avoidance of plagiarism is critical, whereby the use of others' published (or unpublished) work without attributing permission and presenting it as your own is deemed poor practice. As an editor and author, the importance of seeking copyright and permission clearance from sources remains paramount. A good reference of a previously published diagram, for instance, will not suffice. If/when seeking to use previous work, appropriate copyright permission and clearance should be sought in order to reuse material from its original source. As an example, whilst I could have sought diagrams from other research texts for this book, it was decided to commission an illustrator for all depictions throughout. These are termed 'original' and thus require no formal copyright clearances because they remain unique to this book and not elsewhere. For future use, however, prospective authors will require appropriate copyright clearance to whom they belong, in this case CRC Press – the publisher of this book! A well-timed illustration and 'figure' is presented below depicting the concept of 'salami publication' (Elsevier, 2019). The 'salami publication' concept is based on the notion that a single research study/process that creates multiple manuscripts artificially increases the publication volume, as illustrated by Figure 4.1.

This is an interesting concept and one that needs to be monitored, but one, in my view that requires a sensible approach. Clearly, for someone undertaking a BSc honours project, it is expected to lead to a single output in a respectable radiography or other academic journal. For someone embarking onto a PhD, however, which is expected to play a greater part in adding to the evidence base, should by definition, publish 4–5 empirical outputs. Whilst there is no 'set' amount, there is a potential paradox concerning the 'value' of a doctorate, i.e., number of publications and what may be considered 'salami slicing'. As an embryonic researcher reading this, the '1–2–3 rule' offers the anticipation that a BSc (Hons) student could publish one paper, an MSc student, two papers and finally a PhD, a minimum of three

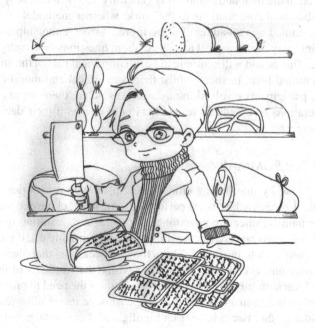

FIGURE 4.1   Depict of the concept of 'salami slicing' in academic dissemination.

papers – this remains a requirement for PhD by publication for some institutions internationally, others requiring 4. This perspective at the very least opens a discussion, accompanied with some 'goal setting' amongst students seeking to publish their work. It does not seek to prescribe the exact number of outputs, as researchers themselves need to work in the ethical context that seeks to publish, but clearly prevent inflation.

Overall, if researchers are acting in an ethical manner, whereby authors are clearly citing and signposting to previous outputs within a manuscript (whilst also clearly highlighting this in an accompanying cover letter), it is a decision for the editors and/or reviewers if new empiricism outweighs the notion of 'incremental salami slicing'. For me, if the theme or evidence is opposed or disproportionate to previously published works from the same study, this clearly benefits the existing evidence base, which may lead to greater impact within our community. Further, other challenges whereby journals have maximum word limit of 4000 words can be problematic for qualitative researchers, especially where descriptive data are presented. If authors, however, are seen to be misleading editors or other members of the journal it could lead to the retraction of articles. Clearly researchers need to be transparent, honest and accountable in order for the editors to decide its appropriateness both from a methodological and empirical perspective and those works previously published.

Whilst ethical issues surround the practice of data dissemination, there are also ethical considerations when considering the contributors of papers. This is important to consider early in the research phase if inviting or collaborating with peers who will be involved in the final authorship. It is generally accepted that only authors who have made substantial contributions to the work, whether methodological or empirical, should be named as a co-author. Furthermore, correct authorship is important to maintain the integrity of the work if any subsequent questions or investigations about the work arise. This is, and will continue to be, an important part of the ethical process and hence identified here. In short, whilst there are ethical and moral concerns that impact on the participants involved in any study, as noted, there are also ethical and moral considerations to uphold as researchers continue with their decision-making throughout a career.

4.6   CHAPTER SUMMARY

This chapter began by introducing ethical principles from a historical perspective. Whilst unethical research has been performed and still acknowledged, these will continue to remain significant cornerstones in our history, resulting in a number of guidance and policy. As researchers we must consider our ethical and moral duty, not only to participants, but to ourselves. There may be occasions that place ourselves in challenging situations, even hostile ones. Thus whilst the emphasis of this chapter is framed around research subjects, we should not dismiss the need to protect ourselves. Whilst the former has been a focus of this chapter due to its significance for research ethics committees, other issues have been highlighted. For instance, not only are ethical considerations necessary prior data collection, but also for monitoring, observing and responding to challenges that arise in the field. Lastly, this chapter focuses on the dissemination phase by discussing what is meant by salami slicing, and how it can be avoided. Ethics does not take place in a vacuum, it is the ongoing set of virtues and practices that guide our behaviours and attitudes to emerging situations. For new researchers looking to begin empirical work, ethical considerations allow you to act in a manner that seeks to improve the care and outcome of participants and self. By learning and reflecting on previous methodological experiences, such as those presented here, we can continuously shape our radiography ethics in order to enhance the health and wellbeing of participants.

KEY TERMS

Anthropomorphic: is the attribution of human traits or conditions, such as tissue in an anthropomorphic X-ray phantom, but is a non-human entity.

Dissemination: is a term used to action or spreading something, which in the case of research is scientific information via publication.

Falsification: is the act of falsifying information from a research project. It can also be used to 'falsify' a theory via the rejection of the null hypothesis in experimental research.

Incognito: is the term used when individuals want to do something and not be recognized. Going incognito means hiding your true identity and is a common tactic for covert researchers.

Nuremberg trials: a series of military tribunals held after World War II by the Allied forces under international law. The trails prosecuted prominent members of those who participated in the Holocaust and other war crimes.

Participant information sheet: is a document that explains the research project to potential participants in order to invite them into the study. This is an essential accompanying document with the consent form, which participants sign prior to beginning in a research study.

Placebo: is a substance or treatment which is deigned to have no effect and thus may deceive the participant in a clinical experiment.

Positionality: is the social and political lens in which our identity, class, gender, sexuality influences and potentially biases alter decision making.

Privacy: is our ability to seclude ourselves of information about oneself. If something is private to a person, it usually means that something is inherently special or sensitive to them.

Protocols: is the procedure or practice of recruiting and then performing research as detailed in an ethics application.

Self-determine: is the concept of being able to determine for oneself without any external influence or pressure.

Social anthropological: is the study of ways in which people behave and live in different social and cultural settings. In different societies, different cultures emerge and this is the same for professional cultures, such as radiography or any other health related field.

EXERCISES AND STUDY QUESTIONS

1   When considering ethical aspects to your related study, perhaps list some features which you feel could potentially impede your participants, or put them at risk. At this stage, you can think broadly and whilst some of your ideas may not be appropriate, after careful discussion with you research supervisors you will be able to focus these considerations.

2   Consider perhaps the research method you intend to use and where this will take place. In response to this, think about consensual practices, for instance, will 'informed consent' be the only necessary practice of consenting individuals during your research process? Can verbal consent be used or could there be scenarios whereby consent will be difficult to collect?

3   Establish your research group early into your research. Regardless of the level of study, consider who your colleagues are in order to support you along the way, but to whom will make valuable contributions to your project in terms of authorship when submitting for publication.

REFERENCES

Ashcroft, A., Dawson, A., Draper, H., and McMillan, J. (2007) *Principles of Health Care Ethics*. West Sussex: Wiley & Sons.

Bailey, C.A. (1996) *A Guide to Field Research*. California: Sage.

Data Protection Act (2018) *The Data Protection Act*. Online, Available at: www.gov.uk/data-protection (Accessed: 08/07/2021).

Dimond, B. (2002) *Legal Aspects of Radiography and Radiology*. Oxford: Blackwell Science.

Elsevier (2019) *FACTSHEET: Salami Slicing*. Online [Available at]: https://www.elsevier.com/__data/assets/pdf_file/0011/653888/Salami-Slicing-factsheet-March-2019.pdf (Accessed: 08/03/2021).

Field, M.J. and Behrman, R.E. (2004) *Ethical Conduct of Clinical Research involving Children*. Washington (DC): National Academies Press (US).

Hammersley, M. (1998) *Reading Ethnographic Research*. 2nd Edn. Wesley Longman: London.

Hayre, C.M. (2016) Radiography observed: an ethnographic study exploring contemporary radiographic practice. Ph.D. Thesis. Canterbury Christ Church University. Faculty of Health and Wellbeing.

Hayre, C.M. and Hackett, P.M.W. (2020) *Handbook of Ethnography in Healthcare Research*. New York: Routledge.

Hayre, C.M., Jeffery, C., and Bungay, H. (2020) Do lead-rubber aprons always limit ionising radiation to radiosensitive organs? *Radiography,* 26 (4), pp. e264–e269.

Jotkowitz, A. (2008) The Holocaust and medical ethics: The voices of the victims. *Journal of Medical Ethics*. 34(1), pp. 869–870.

Kingori, P. and Gerrets, R. (2016) Morals, morale and motivations in data fabrication: Medical research fieldworker's views and practices in two Sub-Saharan African contexts. *Social Science & Medicine*. 166(1), pp. 150–159.

Lawton, J., Hallowell, N., Snowdon, C., Norman, J.E., Carruthers, K., and Denison, F.C. (2017). Written versus verbal consent: a qualitative study of stakeholder views of consent procedures used at the time of recruitment into a peripartum trail conducted in an emergency setting. *BMC Medical Ethics*. 18(36), pp. 1–13.

Mata, R.C., Cardes, A., and Lora, F. (2016) Chapter 5: Good Clinical Practice in Nonprofit Institutions. In *Guide to Cell Therapy GxP*, pp. 177–229. https://www.sciencedirect.com/science/article/pii/B978012803115500005X?via%3Dihub

Petre, M. and Rugg, G. (2004) *The Unwritten Rules of PhD Research.* 2nd Edn. Berkshire: Open University Press.

Petticrew, M., Semple, S., Hilton, S., Creely, KS., Eadie, D., Ritchie, D., Ferrel, C., Christopher, Y., and Hurley, F. (2007) Covert observation in practice: lessons from the evaluation of the prohibition of smoking in public places in Scotland. *BMC Public Health.* 204, pp. 1–8.

Pole, C. and Morrison, M. (2003) *Ethnography for Education.* Berkshire: Open University Press.

Saks, M. and Allsop, J. (2010) *Researching Health – Qualitative, Quantitative and Mixed Method*, Los Angeles: Sage.

Shepherd, M. (2007) *Appraising and Using Social Research in the Human Services – An introduction for Social Work and Health Professionals*, London: Kinsley.

Weindling, P., von Villiez, A., Loewenau, A., and Farron, N. (2016) The victims of unethical human experiments and coerced research under National Socialism. *Endeavour.* 40(1), pp.1–6.

World Health Organization (2021) *Nuremberg Code Turns 60.* Online [Available at]: www.who.int/bulletin/volumes/85/8/07-045443/en/ (Accessed: 07/03/2021).

World Medical Association (2021) *Medical Ethics Manual – Manual for physicians about the role of ethics in medicine.* Online [Available at]: www.wma.net/what-we do/education/medical-ethics-manual/ (Accessed: 07/03/2021).

5 Quantitative Approaches for Radiography

Xiaoming Zheng

5.1 INTRODUCTION

This chapter presents concepts and applications of quantitative research in radiologic science and technology from the author's perspective. It begins with the author's understanding of scientific research in natural and social sciences and the rationale for quantitative research in the interdisciplinary field of radiography. X-ray experiments using imaging systems (computed tomography and radiographic imaging systems) and their related equipment are frequently being carried out in dealing with technical challenges. We will show some X-ray experiments using state-of-the-art equipment and following national and international standards. Non-experimental methodologies are used in dealing with patients where direct experiments on patients are either impractical or unethical. We will show some non-experimental studies including nuclear cardiac imaging and mathematical analysis. Existing data from all sources (published and unpublished) can be mathematically (statistically) analyzed for the benefit of patients. Radiographers are participants and users of epidemiology studies using X-ray imaging technologies. Clinical trials of pharmaceutical drugs, devices or clinical procedures are extremely valuable for people's health. Randomized controlled trials are the most powerful experimental studies on human subjects. In practice, less-stringent clinical studies than randomized controlled trials are often being carried out and these studies are making important contributions to the body of scientific knowledge. We will show our clinical studies on a personalized imaging technique that reduces doses to patients without compromising diagnostic image quality.

5.2 RATIONALE FOR QUANTITATIVE APPROACHES

The purpose of scientific research is to create knowledge about a phenomenon either in the natural world or human society. Scientific knowledge refers to the understanding of the causal relationships between elements of a natural phenomenon or natural laws that govern the world we live in. If the causal relationship between elements of the natural phenomenon can only be expressed by way of description, it is termed qualitative knowledge and the methods of finding such qualitative knowledge are called qualitative research. Conversely, if the causal relationships can be expressed in

DOI: 10.1201/9780367559311-5

mathematical forms (equations), it is called natural laws and the methods of finding these relationships are termed quantitative research. Values and numbers can be used in mathematical equations to predict the behaviour of natural systems. Using numbers and values in scientific studies is part of quantitative research. The quantitative predictions from mathematical equations are generally expected to be accurate enough for practical purposes. Otherwise, these relationships may be considered qualitative descriptions because the uncertainties of predictions are too large to be used in practice. In studying natural phenomena, it is often a challenge to establish a quantitative relationship between elements of a phenomenon. A qualitative description is thus the first step in establishing a quantitative relationship between variables, either in the natural or social sciences. Qualitative research is prevalent in social science, where there is a large amount of uncertainty and in natural science, where the phenomenon is a complex natural system.

Knowledge of science can be used to improve the world we live in and people's health. When scientific knowledge is applied to improve the natural world or people's health, we call it applied science or engineering. Understandably, we prefer precise or quantitative knowledge to be applied in practice, rather than a descriptive direction. It is a fact of life that quantitative causal knowledge is not always available for people in practice like radiographers. This creates challenges for clinical practitioners in applying descriptive knowledge to improve everyday practice when quantitative knowledge for a practical problem is not available.

Radiographers work between machines and patients and radiography deals with technology and people. In dealing with technologies, we are in the domain of natural science (physics) and, in dealing with patients, we are in the domain of social science (psychology). We are working in a multi-disciplinary field between natural and social sciences. Our task is to apply the best technologies to maximize benefits and minimize risks to patients. In X-ray radiography, we expose patients with X-rays and create images for clinical diagnosis that benefit patients in their health management. There is a risk that X-rays can harm patients and health workers if they are not properly protected. For the benefit of patients, we would like to produce the highest possible image quality for accurate diagnosis but the lowest possible X-ray exposure to protect them from the risk of cancer. How to achieve this in clinical practice is a challenge. If one only tells you that the diagnostic image quality is proportional to the radiation dose to patients, or the higher the radiation dose, the higher the image quality for diagnosis, what should you do? You may ask what dose you should prescribe to achieve an optimal image quality for a patient's diagnosis. A qualitative description between image quality and radiation dose to patients is not good enough for minimizing the radiation dose to patients while maintaining the highest image quality for diagnosis. We need a quantitative relationship between the diagnostic image quality and radiation dose to patients.

To establish a quantitative relationship between the image quality and radiation dose to patients, we need to measure image qualities and radiation doses. Radiation doses can be measured using dosimeters and dose measurement is in the domain of natural science. However, diagnostic image quality is a problematic element or variable that is not well defined. Diagnostic image quality is clinical task-dependent and involves human observers – the radiologists. The measurement of image quality is in the domain of social science. Perhaps, the receiver operating characteristic (ROC) assessment (Zheng, et al. 2003; Mets, 2006) or the area under the ROC curve A_z can be considered the best index for measuring image quality, but ROC study is tedious and requires ground truth. Furthermore, every clinical task (anatomic regions and clinical indications) has to be individually studied, which is an enormous, if not impossible, task. On the other hand, we may ask human observers (radiologists) to rank image qualities using a Likert scale based on various image quality criteria such as European image quality criteria (European Commission, 1996; Zheng, Kim and Yang, 2016). This is called a visual grading scale (VGS) study of image quality (Zheng, Kim and Yang, 2016). The Likert scale used in a VGS study is the same as the Likert scale used in education or business research (Sekarran, 2003; Cohen, Manion and Morrison, 2007). The problems of using a VGS for measuring diagnostic image quality are (1) simple arithmetic on the VGS numbers is inappropriate because they are in an ordinal scale; (2) different researchers may use different image quality criteria; (3) there are large variations among human observers. This highlights the difficulties of defining and measuring a complex variable such as diagnostic image quality or abstract elements of a phenomenon to establish a quantitative relationship between them.

5.3 X-RAY EXPERIMENTAL DESIGNS

In radiography, we are dealing with X-ray equipment and patients. Your research questions are likely linked to the X-ray equipment you are using and the patients in your care. There are so many clinical questions we wish to answer, either related to patients or equipment. We have already mentioned the question of minimizing radiation doses to patients while maximizing image quality for diagnosis. We found that we need to first solve the problem of defining image quality because image quality is not well defined and there are many ways of assessing image quality, as discussed above. In doing so, we create a series of sub-questions to be answered before answering the original question. Research involves answering a series of questions – that is why we often call it a research project or program. Medical physicists may measure an image's spatial resolution, noise and contrast to noise ratio as image quality indexes. These indexes are important in assessing X-ray equipment or an imaging system's performance because they have consequences for the radiologists' diagnostic decisions. On the other hand, diagnostic image quality is clinically task-dependent and the image quality index must include clinical outcomes. Physical parameters of spatial resolution, contrast resolution and noise are only part of the total image quality variable. Using physical image quality parameters alone is not good enough for the research question of radiation dose and image quality optimization.

Research design is a research plan to be executed. The design of X-ray experiments is dependent on your research question or sub-question related to your original research question. Your research question must be clearly defined either in answering the primary question or a sub-question. Taking image quality and radiation dose optimization as an example, not only does image quality need to be defined and measured, the radiation dose to patients must also be defined and measured. Direct measurements of radiation doses on patients are impractical, so we use various phantom measures instead. Radiation doses to patients are derived from these phantom measurements under various clinical imaging (or radiotherapy) conditions. For example, doses to CT patients are derived from the dose measurements of CT dose phantoms under various imaging parameters such as the X-ray tube's peak voltage (kVp) and its filament current in milliamperes per second (mAs). Doses to patients in radiographic imaging are derived from the entrance skin (surface) dose (ESD) measurements of an anthropomorphic phantom under various kVp and mAs, as well as the X-ray tube to patient distance or source to object distance (SOD). We know that radiation dose is dependent on the X-ray tube's peak voltage, the filament current and the duration of the exposure. The dose delivered to a patient is also dependent on the distance of the X-ray tube to the patient, the location within the patient's body and the patient's body size. These dependencies or relationships between doses and exposure parameters (kVp, mAs, SOD, etc.) need to be determined and measured to study the image quality responses from various exposures (doses) because doses are dependent on these exposure parameters.

Before designing an X-ray experiment, we should review the literature and international standards for these dose measurements. Some of the experimental data published by international authorities can be used directly and some of the published experimental results in peer-reviewed journals can be critically assessed and used for our study (Aichinger et al., 2004; Compagnone, Pagan and Bergamini, 2005). These can save our experiments or narrow them down to the critical experimental data that we must acquire ourselves. We may have to repeat the experiments published in the literature to complement the published data or remove any inconsistencies of the published data. In our image quality and radiation dose optimization project, we took the published experimental data from the British National Radiation Protection Board to measure the body size effect (Hart et al., 2000) and peer-reviewed experimental measurements on dose versus image quality as reference data for the correlation between image quality and dose (Compagnone, Pagan and Bergamini, 2005). Critical analysis of the published data suggested that the doses delivered to patients at a depth from the body's surface are proportional to the mAs, which is the same as that at the body's surface but appears to have a different power (exponent) to the kVp from that at the body's surface (Aichinger et al., 2004). Determining the dose output exponent of kVp to the body's depth (a location within the body) thus becomes a critical question because we are interested in doses delivered to the body of patients. It is for this sub-question that we designed an X-ray experiment in measuring the dose power (exponent) to the kVp within the body (depth from the body surface) (Zheng, Nardi and Murray, 2017). The outcome of this experiment may not be answering the original question directly. However, it is a key sub-question in answering the original question of determining the optimal imaging parameters (kVp, mAs) for the optimal image quality and radiation dose to patients.

We can design our experiment in detail once the research objectives are clear. We need an X-ray imaging system, a body phantom and a dosimeter. Ideally, the X-ray imaging system should be state-of-the-art and provide us with the capability of varying kVp and mAs, etc., so that we can produce different doses by varying these imaging parameters. Standard phantoms such as the CT dose should be used so that the measured results can be compared with the measured data in the literature. The standard dosimeter, such as an ionizing chamber, can be used. It should be calibrated in national or international laboratories to ensure the reliability and validity of the measured data. It should also be remembered that research is to find new knowledge or explore the unknown. Using existing equipment and repeating others' experiments may not always create new knowledge. One has to be creative and prepared to go beyond using current standard equipment and experiment with something that no one has done before. For instance, anthropomorphic phantoms are commonly used to measure entrance surface doses of the phantom in radiographic imaging. Patients' effective organ doses are calculated (i.e., Monte Carlo simulations) from these measured entrance surface doses. The anthropomorphic phantoms can be used for our purpose, provided that we have these phantoms in our lab together with the dosimeters that can be inserted into the body of the phantom. On the other hand, CT dose phantoms and ionizing dosimeters are standard equipment for CT dose measurements. The CT dose phantom has never been used for measuring doses in radiographic imaging. However, it is a good phantom for our purpose in measuring both the entrance and exit surface doses, as well as doses at the body centre. The benefits of using this phantom for both CT and radiographic dose measurements are that the measured results from both imaging modalities can be compared and a united formulism can be established for both CT and radiographic imaging (Zheng, Nardi and Murray, 2017; Zheng, 2017a).

In designing X-ray experiments, the required equipment may not always be available. You need to consider alternatives or build them yourself. For example, we need a water phantom with holes that can hold different tissue materials (Zheng et al., 2020). The electron density phantom from CRIS is a solid water phantom with 17 holes to hold different inserts of tissue materials. CRIS provided 17 inserts of different tissue materials to fill these holes. However, in our study, we would like to insert one tissue material into one hole at a time while filling the rest of the holes with water equivalent inserts. This is to remove the interference on the tissue's CT number from the neighbouring tissue materials. The solutions could be to purchase solid water inserts from the company or to make these water inserts ourselves. Our simple solution is to fill these holes with water balloons (filled with tap water). It is an effective, convenient and cheap solution.

5.4 NON-EXPERIMENTAL DESIGNS

The difference between experimental and non-experimental design is whether or not the phenomenon's independent variables are manipulated in the study. Scientific knowledge or the causal relationship between dependent and independent variables can be established by either manipulating the independent variables, such as kVp and mAs in our experimental X-ray study, or by observing (measuring) the responses of dependent variables on independent variables without manipulating the independent variables, such as the correlation between body sizes and patients' doses using data from the British Radiation Protection Board (Hart et al., 2000). Natural phenomena are generally complicated and existing facts or data are either insufficient, inconsistent or not available to provide the causal relationship between variables. Scientific progress is indeed heavily dependent on experimental evidence for support. This is why the experimental study is such a robust methodology in research. Scientists set up experiments and artificially vary (or manipulate) the variables and measure (observe) the responses of dependent variables to establish or validate the causal relationships between variables. These experiments can be carried out in laboratories or within human society under varied settings, although societal experiments on human subjects are much harder to perform. True experimental studies on human subjects have well-defined protocols and procedures as defined in randomized controlled trials (Friedman et al., 2015). Some studies on human subjects can only be classified as quasi-experimental because the subjects' recruitment and group assignment are not randomized in the study design. There are many cases where the manipulations of the independent variables are either impractical or impossible, such as ethics considerations on human subjects. In these cases, alternative measurements (observations) without manipulating the independent variables should be considered. Non-experimental studies are equally important to the experimental approach in research and, in some cases, they are the only way to achieve the desired outcomes.

In nuclear cardiac imaging, caffeine has been shown to induce false-negative ^{201}Tl myocardial perfusion using the pharmacologic stressor dipyridamole (Zheng and Williams, 2002). The question is, how much serum caffeine level will induce a false-negative ^{201}Tl myocardial perfusion? It is not good to manipulate patients' serum caffeine levels by injections to determine the caffeine level for false-negative imaging. We should seek a non-experimental research design. If the serum caffeine level for a false-negative ^{201}Tl myocardial perfusion is established, then, what is the best indicator for the serum caffeine level? It is not good to have a blood caffeine test for every patient undergoing myocardial imaging. We should seek alternatives. In our study, we measured patients' blood pressures and heart rates and the serum caffeine levels of 36 patients before and after the infusion of dipyridamole stressor. There is no correlation between blood pressure and serum caffeine levels but there is an inverse relationship between the heart rate increase and caffeine levels. We predicted that a less than 5% heart rate increase or a larger than 2 mg/L serum caffeine level would produce false-negative ^{201}Tl myocardial perfusion images (Zheng and Williams, 2002). This example shows that the non-experimental design does not have to be non-experimental measurement. It is the non-manipulation of the independent variables, such as non-manipulation of patients' caffeine levels by injecting caffeine into the patients. We can see that the correlation between caffeine levels and heart rates is established without manipulating the blood caffeine levels. It suggested that the heart rate could be an indicator for false-negative ^{201}Tl myocardial perfusion imaging.

Mathematically speaking, minimizing a radiation dose to patients while maintaining the highest image quality for patients' diagnosis in X-ray imaging is an optimization operation, provided that the relationship between the dose and image quality is known. It would be a simple mathematical operation of differentiation on the image quality as a function of the dose. We found that the relationships between image quality and dose as evidenced in the literature, are not consistent, as linear (Zheng, Kim and Yang, 2016), logarithmic (Zheng, 2016a, 2017b) and logistic functions (Zheng et al., 2014) have all been reported. The reason for this inconsistency could be partly because the image quality index is a complicated index and partly because of the inaccuracy of dose measurements at low doses (Zheng, 2016b). Considering all possible functions for the relationship and the measured dose expression within patients, we have derived a general equation that guides radiographers in the optimal selection of image parameters kVp and mAs based on patient's body thickness (Zheng, 2017a, 2018). Under this general equation, radiation exposures can be prescribed individually for personalized dose prescriptions in CT and radiographic imaging. This general equation can be implemented in the imaging systems to replace all the empirical 'rules of thumb' such as the 15% and 2 kV/cm rules in clinical practice (Al-Balool and Newman, 1998; Targett and McLean, 2001; Allen et al., 2013), or exposure charts such as fixed and variable kilo-voltage systems as described in radiographic textbooks (Carlton and Adler, 2006). More importantly, by using a personalized exposure prescription, the doses to patients can be reduced significantly without compromising diagnostic image quality. For example, under a constant kVp, the exposure mAs can be reduced by half in comparison with the current manufacturers' recommendations if the patient's body thickness is increased by 1 cm in radiographic imaging (Williams et al., 2007). For CT imaging of children, it suggests a lower kVp should be used with a prescribed less mAs increase, which will significantly reduce the dose to children (Zheng, 2018).

The above discussion suggests that mathematical analysis can be one of the powerful non-experimental research designs. It can uncover hidden causal relationships among variables of a phenomenon. In another example, experimental data have shown that CT numbers (in the Hounsfield unit) vary from patient to patient depending on their body size (Hsieh, 2015; Zheng et al., 2020). This affects both quantitative patient diagnosis and radiation dose delivery to patients in radiotherapy (Inaniwa, Tashima and Kanematsu, 2018). Beam hardening of polychromatic X-rays is believed to be the cause (Hsieh, 2015). When polychromatic X-rays pass through a patient's body, the lower energies part of the X-ray energy spectrum will have higher attenuation coefficients. Therefore, more X-rays at lower energies are attenuated than that from the higher energies part of the X-ray spectrum. As a result, the averaged energy of the transmitted X-rays is higher (hardening) than the average energy of the X-rays before the transmission. This would lead to a reduced attenuation coefficient, or CT number in the Hounsfield unit after X-rays pass through a depth within the tissue. This is termed beam hardening. However, experimental results showed that CT numbers (attenuation coefficients) are increased if the same tissue is moved from a location to a deeper location within the body (Zheng et al., 2020). To understand why tissues' CT numbers (in the Hounsfield unit) change from different body sizes and depths within the body, we have carried out a theoretical analysis of X-ray interactions with bulk water using the Boltzmann transport equation. It reveals that Rayleigh scatterings play an important role. A correction scheme has been established for the variation of CT numbers from different body sizes and depths within the body (Zheng et al., 2020).

A systemic review with statistical analysis or meta-analysis is non-experimental research by design (Bruce, Pope and Stanistreet, 2018). It is similar to the mathematical analysis discussed above, except for statistical analysis on some independent studies. Scientific research is a joint effort of many independent scientists. Different researchers may face different challenges either from limitations of resources and equipment or by the nature of the research question itself. An important research question may attract many researchers but different researchers may produce different results, which render their findings inconclusive or even incorrect. A systemic review and statistical analysis of the studies about the same research question can help to reach a better conclusion with higher confidence (Bruce, Pope and Stanistreet, 2018). It should be noted that a systemic review is not the same as a literature review for a research proposal. A literature review for a research proposal is aimed at identifying gaps or problems for further study. A systematic review is to critically analyse the existing data on the research question and reach better conclusions or develop a better solution at a higher level of confidence. There are standard steps in designing a systemic review study, such as identify data sources (published and non-published), study selection criteria (quality of the research), statistical analysis methods (Funnel diagram, Forest tree), etc. (Bruce, Pope and Stanistreet, 2018). For example, there is evidence that a reduction of the hippocampus volume is linked to Alzheimer's disease (AD). Researchers are interested in finding out if the hippocampus volume can be used as a biomarker to predict the onset of Alzheimer's disease or an earlier indication of possible conversion into Alzheimer's from a mild cognition impairment (MCI) (Shi et al., 2009). Magnetic resonance imaging is an excellent tool in measuring hippocampus volumes. Many studies are using MRI T1 weighted images to measure the hippocampus volumes of AD patients and MCI patients. Different numbers of patients (generally small numbers) and statistical analysis have been used in different studies. Published data results are not consistent; some areas of inconsistency include the volumes for the MCI patients and symmetry between the left and the right hippocampus volumes. A systematic review has been carried out which provided improved statistics and conclusions (Shi et al., 2009). A systematic review is non-experimental research by design and should be treated as just one of the many studies on the same research question.

5.5 EPIDEMIOLOGY

Epidemiology is the study of the distribution, detriments and frequency of diseases in the human population (Bruce, Pope and Stanistreet, 2018). One of the main purposes of epidemiology is to determine the broader causes of diseases so that policymakers can take preventive measures to protect the population and curb the disease. Research methods in epidemiology can be descriptive (qualitative) or quantitative. Quantitative methods such as surveys, case-control studies, cohort studies, intervention studies or natural experiments can be used (Bruce, Pope and Stanistreet, 2018). Each of these methodologies has advantages and disadvantages. The choice of a method is dependent on the research question and the resources available to you. Disease survey screening, such as breast or lung cancer, using X-ray imaging is one method used in epidemiology studies. A screening program is designed to assess people in the population who are at risk for disease and classify them as having either a high risk or low chance of actually having the disease at an earlier stage so that those of high risk can be referred to have a definitive assessment and those with low risk can be reassured. Survey screening, in general, requires repeated examinations of a large number of healthy people. The screening test needs to be accurate with simplicity, low cost, safety and acceptability. A screening survey is a substantial and demanding task and the program itself should be evaluated (Bruce, Pope and Stanistreet, 2018).

One of the criteria in evaluating a screen survey program is the validity of the disease screening. Several indexes can measure the validity, such as sensitivity, specificity, predictive values, accuracy, etc. Sensitivity is defined as the true positive fraction and specificity is the true negative fraction. The problem in using only sensitivity or specificity is that the observers' (radiologists') decision criteria can vary. If a decision threshold is very strict, then some true positive cases will be missed and if a decision threshold is too lax, then some negative cases will be classified as positive. The best method is the receiver operating characteristic (ROC) study (Mets, 2006) – this method combines the sensitivity and specificity into one index called the area under the curve, Az. The ROC curve is a plot of the sensitivity in the y-axis versus (1-specificity) x-axis where the sensitivities and specificities are measured on several decision thresholds (varied strictness and laxness). The ROC study is a gold standard method in radiology that can be used to evaluate many different performances, including the performance of radiologists themselves (Zheng et al., 2003; Mets, 2006).

The results of epidemiology studies have been used for radiation protection purposes (ICRP, 2007). One responsibility of radiographers in practice is to minimize the radiation dose to patients and protect medical radiation workers and the public from radiation exposure. To make informed decisions, we would like to know the relationship between health risk (tissue responses) and radiation dose so that an optimal decision can be made in balancing the benefit with the risk of harm to patients, workers and the public. This is similar to the dose and image quality optimization problem discussed earlier. At high radiation dose levels, such as those used in radiotherapy, we can measure the tissues' responses with reasonable certainty. This is termed a deterministic response. However, at low dose levels, such as those used in medical imaging, there is considerable uncertainty in the measurement of the tissues' responses. This large uncertainty is termed a stochastic response. In the low-dose regime, dose measurement itself involves a large degree of uncertainty, even if the dosimeter has been calibrated to national or international standard laboratories (Zheng, 2016b). The focus of radiation protection is mainly on the low dose regime and the large uncertainties in measuring the doses and tissues' responses made it difficult to determine the relationship between health risk and radiation doses. The International Commission on Radiation Protection (ICRP) therefore turned to epidemiology studies for evidence in establishing its recommendations on radiation protection policy. Data from any large-scale epidemiology studies are best for this purpose, but studies at smaller scales can also be beneficial.

One of the most comprehensive epidemiology studies of radiation exposures on human health is the Japanese Life Span Study (LSS) of A-bomb survivors' children. This is a longitudinal cohort study in design. Other radiation-exposed populations have also been used by the ICRP (2007), such as (1) patients with therapeutic or diagnostic exposure to radiation; (2) workers exposed to radiation in the course of their jobs such as radiographers or radiologists; (3) persons with environmental exposures such as from the fallout of the Chernobyl incident. Studies of categories 1 and 2 may be classified as a cohort or cohort-control in research design and the study of the Chernobyl incident may be classified as a natural experiment. It should be noted that interventional experiment design can also be used in epidemiology studies (Bruce, Pope and Stainistreet, 2018). For example, based on evidence, we may implement a radiation protection measure such as wearing a pair of protective glasses during patient positioning. We can study the impact of the interventional measure of wearing protective glasses on radiographers' eye diseases rates.

It is worth noting that the relationship between the health risk and radiation exposure depends on the definition of the health risk. Like diagnostic image quality, health risk is a complicated index and it can vary depending on researchers' consensus in capturing the fundamental factors of people's health. Many factors can be part of the health risk index, such as mortality rate, life expectancy shortening and quality of life. Quality of life itself can have many factors. The definition of health risk by the ICRP has evolved over the years. Despite all the best efforts in establishing the health risk and dose relationship at low doses, the recommended linear no-threshold model is still debatable (ICRP, 2007). Research on approving and disapproving the no-threshold model in radiation protection is ongoing.

5.6   CLINICAL TRIAL METHODOLOGY

The World Health Organization (WHO) defines a clinical trial as

> a type of research that studies new tests and treatments and evaluates their effects on human health outcomes. People volunteer to take part in clinical trials to test medical interventions including drugs, cells and other biological products, surgical procedures, radiological procedures, devices, behavioral treatments and preventive care.

(WHO, 2021)

Most people are familiar with trials of pharmaceuticals or drugs where the results of large-scale clinical trials, such as Covid-19 vaccines, are frequently reported in the media. By the WHO's definition, clinical trials are much broader than the trials of pharmaceutical drugs. They include clinical devices and procedures or clinical protocols. A clinical trial is also called a clinical investigation, clinical evaluation or simply clinical research.

Clinical research can be categorized by experimental or observational studies. Experimental studies can be controlled or uncontrolled trials and controlled experimental studies can be randomized or non-randomized. Observational studies can be divided into cohort or case-control studies or cross-sectional studies. Clinical investigation can also be classified based on the timing of data collection: retrospective or prospective. For retrospective studies, one collects and analyses patients' data that already exist (backward in time) to answer the research questions. For prospective studies, we collect participants' data forward in time (no data at the starting time) to determine causal associations. In cross-sectional studies, we examine exposure and outcome simultaneously at a particular time without looking forward or backward. In case-control studies, investigators compare exposed with non-exposed (control) groups. In cohort studies, investigators compare subsequent incidences of disease among groups distinguished by one or more exposures. Comparative clinical trials are prospective cohort studies that compare treatments assigned to patients by the researchers. A more restrictive definition of a clinical trial is a 'prospective study comparing the effects and value of intervention (s) against a control in human beings' (Friedman et al., 2015). In this definition, the study has to be (1) prospective; (2) interventional (experimental); (3) controlled (a control group against which the interventional group is compared) and (4) involve human beings. The prospective randomized case-controlled clinical trials are the preferred method for evaluating medical interventions. In social science such as psychology, business or education, randomized controlled experiments on human subjects are considered true experimental studies. Some less-stringent study designs may be termed quasi-experimental studies [5], such as non-randomized control studies.

In radiographic imaging, clinical investigations can be of any new contrast agents, devices including new imaging systems and procedures including new imaging protocols (Zheng, 2002; Zheng et al., 2018). In contrast agent studies, radiographers may focus on contrast effect on image quality and radiation dose to patients, rather than the effects of drugs on disease treatments as in general clinical trials. Most medical devices are developed by R&D companies or manufacturers and radiographers may join their clinical evaluations in practice. The design of clinical trials is centred on safety and efficacy or performance. In clinical trials of both drugs and medical devices, there are several phases or stages. In general, the safety of the drug or device is tested in the earlier phase or initial stage with a small number of subjects. The second phase is to test the efficacy of drugs or performance of devices, again with a small number of subjects. The first and second stages may be combined as a single phase, which is often the case in testing medical devices. The third phase is a large-scale trial that may involve hundreds or thousands of subjects where the safety and efficacy are seriously being tested. The final phase is ongoing monitoring of the safety and efficacy in clinics after the regulator's approval for clinical applications. Phases III and IV may be considered as a single phase, just as phases I and II can be combined as a single phase. However, it is difficult to follow these standard phases or stages for clinical trials of surgical or radiological procedures. Several factors distinguish clinical evaluations of medical procedures from trials of drugs and devices. These include small patient number size, variations in procedural competence, and strong surgeon and patient preference. Different approaches have been used in clinical studies of radiological procedures or imaging protocols.

In our studies of reducing radiation doses to patients while maintaining diagnostic image quality, we have derived a general equation in guiding radiographers on the optimal selection of imaging parameters, such as kVp and mAs, taking an individual patient's body size into account, or personalized exposure prescription

(Zheng, 2017, 2018). These equations suggest that under a constant kVp in radiographic imaging and if the patient's body size is increased by 1 cm, only half of the exposure (mAs) increase is needed compared to that used in current clinical practice (Zheng, 2017). Our next research question was to test these predictions in clinical practice (a clinical study or clinical trial). We designed a prospective clinical study based on the available equipment (a mobile C-arm radiographic system) and patient population (chest imaging and follow-ups) within one university hospital (Zheng et al., 2018). We selected a cohort of patients whose follow-up images were required. The personalized exposure prescriptions were applied during the follow-up imaging so that the patients' initial chest images acted as the controls. An experienced radiologist was blind to the study and reported (evaluated) both initial and follow-up images for a cohort of 42 patients. The radiologist reported no difference between the initial and follow-up images in terms of clinical diagnosis. This result suggests that the personalized exposure prescription scheme effectively reduces the radiation dose to patients while maintaining an accurate patient diagnosis.

Continuing innovation and improvement in clinical practice require many clinical studies before the intended benefits can be transferred to patients and the general population. These innovations can be any new imaging procedures or protocols or computer software to assist radiologists' diagnoses. Many of the current artificial intelligence (AI) algorithms for medical imaging require rigorous clinical trials (tests) before the regulatory authority, such as FDA, can approve their use in clinics. Computer algorithms such as AI software are considered a medical device and their use in clinical practice requires the approval of regulatory authorities, just like other medical devices. As discussed above, clinical trials of devices may have slightly different designs from those involving pharmaceutical drug trials. However, the multiphase randomized controlled trials (RCT) of drugs can serve as the gold standard for all clinical studies. Variations from the RCT standard may be used depending on the research question and available resources.

5.7 CHAPTER SUMMARY

Scientific research aims to create knowledge about the causal relationships among elements of a natural phenomenon. Knowledge can be used to improve the world we live in and people's health. Radiographers work in a multi-disciplinary field of applied science dealing with technologies and patients. Quantitative knowledge is preferred for practical applications in the field of radiography. Radiographers face many challenges every day in carrying out their work. They use research as a tool to find answers for many clinical questions related to people and technology. X-ray experiments using imaging systems (CT and radiographic systems) and their related equipment are frequently being carried out in dealing with technical challenges. In designing X-ray experiments, we are not only following national and international standards and using state-of-the-art equipment, we are being creative and prepared to go beyond conventional practice and procedures. Non-experimental methodologies are used in dealing with patients where direct variable manipulations on patients are either impractical or unethical. We are also applying analytical skills on existing data from all sources (published and unpublished), including local imaging information systems, for the benefit of our patients. We use the results of epidemiology studies for radiation protection of our patients, fellow health workers and the public. We are participants in some epidemiology studies, such as breast or lung disease screenings, using X-ray imaging technologies. Clinical trials of pharmaceutical drugs, devices or clinical procedures are extremely valuable for the benefit of patients. Randomized controlled trials are the most powerful experimental studies on human subjects. The main characteristics of RCT study design are the randomized recruitment of participants and randomized assignment of participants into experiment and control groups. In practice, less-stringent clinical studies than the RCT are often being carried out and these studies are making equally important contributions to the body of scientific knowledge.

KEY TERMS

Causal relationship: exists if the occurrence of the first causes the other. The first event is termed the 'cause' and the second event is termed the 'effect'.

Clinical trial methodology: is a research study that assigns human participants or groups of humans to one or more health-related interventions to evaluate the effects of health outcomes.

Diagnostic image quality: is a measure that seeks to determine the quality of a radiography image using scales and measures.

Disease screening: is used in medicine as a strategy to look for as-yet-unrecognized conditions or risk markers.

Epidemiology: is the study and analysis of the distribution and patterns of health and disease conditions in defined populations and remains a cornerstone of public health.

Experimental research: is a procedure carried out to support, refute or validate a hypothesis. Experiments provide insight into cause-and-effect by demonstrating what outcome occurs when a particular variable is manipulated.

Health risk: is a risk assessment and a widely used tool for screening in the field of health promotion.

Mathematical analysis: deals with the branch of mathematics dealing with limits and related theories including differentiation, integration and measure.

Non-experimental research: lacks the manipulation of an independent variable, random assignment and thus measure variables as they naturally occur in the real world.

Quantitative research: is a research strategy that focuses on quantifying the collection of numerical information and utilizes deductive reasoning to inform empirical outcomes.

Radiation dose: is a measure of ionizing radiation in radiography that patients receive when undergoing radiological procedures. Absorbed dose is measured in gray (Gy) whereas effective dose is measured in Sievert (Sv).

Systematic review: is a type of review that uses repeatable analytical methods to collect, sort and analyse secondary data.

EXERCISES AND STUDY QUESTIONS

1   Define scientific knowledge and applied science.
2   Explain the differences between quantitative and qualitative research approaches.
3   Why is quantitative knowledge preferred in radiography?
4   Explain the differences between experimental and non-experimental research designs.
5   Explain how patients' absorbed radiation doses and effective radiation doses are measured in X-ray CT and radiographic imaging.
6   A manufacturer of radiographic imaging systems provided factory pre-set imaging protocols. Explain how you would apply these pre-set protocols in clinical practice.
7   You are asked to assess the validity of a breast screening program. Please provide a detailed research plan on how to do the assessment.
8   A software company has developed a computer-assisted diagnosis tool. Please explain how to carry out your clinical trial for the software.

REFERENCES

Aichinger, H., Dierker, J., Joite-Barfub, S., and Sabel, M. (2004). *Radiation Exposure and Image Quality in X-Ray Diagnostic Radiology: Physical Principles and Clinical Applications*. Berlin: Springer-Verlag.

Al-Balool, G.S. and Newman, D.L. (1998). The relationships between kV, mAs and the thickness in film-based radiography: 25% and 15% rules. *Radiography*, 4, pp. 129–134.

Allen, E., Hogg, P., Ma, W.K., and Szczepura, K. (2013). Fact or fiction: An analysis of 10 kVp 'rule' in computed radiography. *Radiography*, 19, pp. 223–227.

Bruce, N., Pope, D., and Stanistreet, D. (2018). *Quantitative Methods for Health Research: A Practical Interactive Guide to Epidemiology and Statistics*. 2nd Edn, Hoboken: John Wiley & Sons Ltd.

Carlton, R.R. and Adler, A.M. (2006). *Principles of Radiographic Imaging: An Art and a Science*. 4th Edn. NY: Delmar Cengage Learning

Cohen, L., Manion, L., and Morrison, K. (2007). *Research Methods in Education*. 6th Edn. London: Routledge Taylor and Francis Group.

Compagnone, G., Pagan, L., and Bergamini, C. (2005). Comparison of six phantoms for entrance skin dose evaluation in 11 standard X-ray examinations. *Journal of Applied Clinical Medical Physics*. 6(1), pp. 101–113.

European Commission, (1996). European guidelines on quality criteria for diagnostic radiographic images. Office for Official Publications of European Communities.

Friedman, L.M., Furberg, C.D., DeMets, D.L., Reboussin, D.M., and Granger, C.B. (2015). *Fundamentals of Clinical Trials*. 5th Edn. Heidelberg: Springer.

Hart, D., Wall, B.F., Shrimpton, P.C. and Bungay, D.R. (2000). Reference doses and patient size in paediatric radiology. National Radiological Protection Board Reports (R318). Chilton. UK.

Hsieh, J. (2015). *Computed Tomography: Principles, Design Artefacts and Recent Advances*. Bellingham: SPIE Press.

ICRP. Publication 103. (2007). The 2007 recommendations of the International Commission on Radiological Protection. *Annals of the ICRP*, 37.

Inaniwa, T., Tashima, H. and Kanematsu, N. (2018). Optimal size of a calibration phantom for X-ray CT to convert the Hounsfield units to stopping power ratio in charged particle therapy treatment planning. *Journal of Radiology Research.* 59(2), pp. 216–224.

Mets, C.E. (2006). Receiver operating characteristic analysis: A tool for quantitative evaluation of observer performance and imaging systems. *Journal of the American College of Radiology.* 3, pp. 413–422.

Sekarran, U. (2003). *Research Methods for Business: A Skill-Building Approach.* 4th Edn. New York: John Wiley & Sons, Inc.

Shi, F., Liu, B., Zhou, Y., Yu, C., and Jian, T. (2009). Hippocampal volume and asymmetry in mild cognitive impairment and Alzheimer's disease: Meta-analysis of MRI studies. *Hippocampus.* 19, pp. 1055–1064.

Targett, C., and McLean, D. (2001). Exposure determination: Examining the validity of the 25%/cm rule. *The Radiographer.* 48, pp. 5–8.

WHO. Clinical trials. www.who.int/health-topics/clinical-trials/#tab=tab_1. Accessed on: 22/02/2021.

Williams, M.B., Krupinski, E.A., Strauss, K.J., Breeden, W.K., and Rzeszokarski, M.S. (2007). Digital image quality: Image acquisition. *Journal of the American College of Radiology.* 4, pp. 37–88.

Zheng, X.M. (2002). Detecting regional cerebral blood flow changes in alzheimer's patients after milameline treatment: activation or baseline SPECT? *Journal of Nuclear Medicine Technology.* 30, pp. 115–118.

Zheng, X. (2016a). Attenuation based governing equations for automatic exposure and peak voltage controls in medical X-ray CT imaging. *CT Theory and Applications.* 25(6), pp. 625–632.

Zheng, X. (2016b). Dose correction in medical X-ray imaging at low dose regime. *Journal of Medical Imaging and Health Informatics* 6(7), pp. 1818–1822.

Zheng, X. (2017a). General equations for optimal selection of diagnostic image acquisition parameters in clinical X-ray imaging. *Radiological Physics and Technology.* 10(4), pp. 415–421.

Zheng, X. (2017b). Patient size based guiding equations for automatic mAs and kVp selections in general medical X-ray projection radiography. *Radiation Protection Dosimetry.* 174(4), pp. 545–550.

Zheng, X. (2018). Body size and tube voltage-dependent guiding equations for optimal selection of image acquisition parameters in clinical X-ray imaging. *Radiological Physics and Technology.* 11(2), pp. 212–218.

Zheng, X., Al-Hayek, Y., Cummins, C., Li, X., Nardi, L., Albari, K., Evans, J., Roworth, E., and Seaton, T. (2020). Body size and tube voltage dependent corrections for Hounsfield Unit in medical X-ray computed tomography: Theory and experiments. *Scientific Reports.* 10, pp. 15696.

Zheng, X., Chiang, H.-W., Li, J.-H., Chiang, H.-J., and Lin, L.-H. (2018). Personal exposure prescription method reduces dose in radiography. *Radiological Technology.* 89(5), pp. 435–440.

Zheng, X.M., Gifford, H.C., Pretorius, P.H., and King, M.A. (2003). An observer study of reconstruction strategies for the detection of solitary pulmonary nodules using hybrid NeoTect SPECT images. *IEEE Nuclear Science Symposium and Medical Imaging Conference Record.* 4, pp. 2690–2694.

Zheng, X., Kim, T.M., and Yang, S. (2016). Optimal kVp in chest computed radiography using visual grading scores: A comparison between visual grading characteristics and ordinal regression analysis. *Proceedings of SPIE (Medical Imaging).* 9783, pp. 97836A1–97836A8.

Zheng, X., Nardi, L., and Murray, M. (2017). Size effect on dose output in phantoms of X-ray tubes in medical X-ray imaging. *Biomedical Physics and Engineering Express.* 3:065004.

Zheng, X.M. and Williams, R.C. (2002). On serum caffeine levels after 24 hours abstention: Clinical implications on dipyridamole-thallium-201 myocardial perfusion imaging. *Journal of Nuclear Medicine Technology.* 30, pp. 123–127.

Zheng, X., Kim, T.M., Davidson, R., Lee, S., Shin, C., and Sook Yang, S. (2014). CT X-ray tube voltage optimization and image reconstruction evaluation using visual grading analysis. *Proceedings of SPIE (Medical Imaging).* 9033, pp. 903328.

6 Data Collection in Quantitative Research

Xiaoming Zheng

6.1 INTRODUCTION

This chapter concerns data collection in quantitative research. Data is not knowledge but knowledge creation relies on accurate data. Measurement is central to data collection, which is a multi-step process. The collection of high-quality data is guided by scientific intuition and the use of state-of-the-art or the highest quality instruments. Data collection procedures stipulated in randomized controlled trials (RCT) are a gold standard for clinical investigations. Procedures less stringent than RCT procedures can be considered as quasi-experimental or pilot studies. Questionnaire surveys are a popular non-experimental data collection approach and we have used this method for various radiologic studies. The key to survey studies is the construct of questionnaire items that capture the principal components of the research question. Imaging information systems such as a picture archive and communication system (PACS) and publicly available clinical and imaging databases can be valuable sources of non-experimental data. We have used these databases for various studies, including derivations of various governing equations for optimal selections of imaging parameters in X-ray imaging. Published literature or unpublished data are collected for systematic review studies. Scientific knowledge should be generalizable and knowledge claims must be validated with high confidence.

6.2 MEASUREMENT PROCESS

Scientific measurement is at the centre of quantitative research. It assigns numbers to a system's variables or elements of the phenomenon under study. For example, we use ionizing chambers to measure CT radiation doses and assign a number to the measured quantity (amount) of the dose. For this simple measurement, we need an instrument (ionizing chamber), the element or variable which is the dose, a scale and unit, which is a ratio scale in milligray. Other measurements, such as measuring diagnostic image quality, are not that straightforward. First, diagnostic image quality (element or dependent variable) itself is not well defined. It is clinical task (outcome) dependent. The instrument is the human observer who reads the images. We need a scale to quantize the image quality, such as a Likert scale used in education research

DOI: 10.1201/9780367559311-6

(Cohen, Manion and Morrison, 2007). The Likert scale is different from the ratio scale used in radiation dose (mGy) measurement (Kothari, 2004). The numbers in a Likert scale are called ordinal numbers – number 3 minus number 2 does not equal number 4 minus number 3. If the Likert scale is not accurate in measuring image quality, what is the best index for measuring diagnostic image quality? We can see that scientific measurement can be a complicated task.

The measurement process begins with the research question. We need a clear objective for what we are trying to achieve and the research question has to be specific. In many cases, the measurement is aimed at answering a sub-question of the original question. In the dose and image quality optimization example, the original objective is to reduce the radiation dose to patients while achieving a suitable diagnostic image quality. The original task is to establish the relationship between diagnostic image quality and the radiation dose to patients, so that we can use mathematical operations of optimization to determine the optimal dose and image quality for a diagnosis. To answer the original question, we have to carry out two kinds of measurements: (1) radiation doses to patients and (2) image quality corresponding to the exposed radiation dose. We need clear definitions of the variables of dose and image quality before we can measure them. Dose is defined as the amount of radiation energy deposited to a target per unit mass. Diagnostic image quality is defined as the usefulness for clinical diagnosis. The energy deposited to a target per unit mass is well defined and clear to us, but the clinical 'usefulness' of the quality of an image is an abstract concept. This kind of abstract concept or element of a phenomenon is termed a 'construct' in social science. Defining variables or constructs to be measured is the first step in the measurement process.

The second step is to determine the measurement instrument or develop a construct. A construct is often termed an instrument in disciplines of social science such as business finance. In our dose and image quality optimization example, radiation doses are measured by dosimeters and there are many different types of radiation dosimeters. The type of radiation dosimeter to be used is dependent on availability and suitability for the measurement task. There are standardized equipment and measurement procedures for many specific measurement tasks, such as those formulated by professional bodies, e.g., the American Association of Physicists in Medicine (AAPM). These standard procedures and equipment are recommended because they produce experimental measurements that are generally more reliable than those from non-standard equipment and procedures. Diagnostic image quality, however, is an abstract concept that has many aspects, including factors relating to human observers. There are different ways to formulate the concept of image quality. For example, one can use receiver operating characteristics study (ROC) using human observers' true positive and true negative fractions with varied decision thresholds to determine the outcome (usefulness) of patients' diagnoses (Zheng et al., 2003) or use several image quality criteria such as the visibility of anatomical parts and structures or characteristic features to construct an image quality index (Zheng et al., 2015, 2016). The specific image quality instrument to be used will determine the next step in the data collection process.

The third step is to determine the data items to be measured to answer the research question or the constitutive elements to be included for the construct so that a quantitative value can be assigned to the construct. For example, we measured doses at the entrance and exit surfaces as well as the centre of a body phantom in radiographic imaging; central and peripheral doses of a CT dose phantom in computed tomography (Zheng, Nardi and Murray, 2017). The exit surface doses in radiographic imaging are purposely measured to establish the relationship between the exponent of the kVp and body size at the exit surface. In CT dose measurement, data items at the peripheral and centre of the phantom are used to determine the averaged dose, such as the CT dose index, CTDIv. In our study, the doses measured at the centre of different-sized phantoms are used to determine the size effects (Zheng, Nardi and Murray, 2017). In a different experiment, we need to decide the number of tissue samples and phantom body sizes to be measured in our electron density phantom study (Zheng et al., 2020). The decision on the number of samples is based on the balance between sufficient evidence and the burden on a clinical CT scanner. The number of two phantom sizes was used in our experiment owing to the fact that the phantom company provides only two phantom sizes. For image quality measurement using a visual grading scale, we need to select the major criteria items to be included in the image quality measurement. For example, we may include physical image quality parameters such as overall noise and contrast, and diagnostic relevant items such as anatomical regions of media sternum, parenchyma and bronchus in chest radiographic imaging (Zheng, Kim and Yang, 2016). Careful selection of the criteria items is important as it will impact the research outcome. If we use the area under the curve, Az, of a receiver operating characteristics (ROC) study as the image quality index, we need to decide the number of decision threshold points: one, three or five points (very strict, strict, normal, lax and very lax in the decision criteria) and ask the observers to make their decisions on the images under different decision thresholds. Each of the different decision thresholds means a repeated evaluation of the whole set of images. One can appreciate the workload added on the observers for every increased decision threshold point. In principle, we can construct an ROC curve based on a single optimal decision point, assuming normal distributions of signal and background, but the ROC curve constructed by five decision threshold points should be more accurate than that from the one threshold point. In practice, one needs to balance the accuracy and workload to achieve the desired outcome.

The fourth step is to determine the measurement scale. There are four types of scales in scientific measurements: nominal, ordinal, interval and ratio (Kothari, 2004). A nominal or category scale is an indication of difference only, such as male or female. Assigning a number 1 or 2 to a category does not mean category 1 is less than category 2. An ordinal scale suggests a direction of difference, i.e., if 3>2 and 4>3 then 4>2. However, 3–2 does not equal 4–3. An interval scale represents quantities that have equal units but the number zero does not mean the quantity is zero. It is just another point of measurement. For example, 60°C is 30°C higher than 30°C but it does not mean that 60°C is two times hotter than 30°C. A ratio scale has an absolute zero, i.e., the quantity is zero. Otherwise, a ratio scale is the same as an interval scale. For example, 60°K (Kelvin has an absolute zero degree) is two times hotter than 30°K. Measurements in physics are generally in a ratio or interval scale, such as radiation dose in m milligray but image quality evaluated in a Likert scale is in an ordinal scale. Mathematically, it is inappropriate to average ordinal numbers like the numbers in a ratio scale, but ordinal regression can be used for handling the numbers in an ordinal scale.

The fifth step involves assigning numbers to the system's variables or constructs. In our example, this would involve reading out numbers from the dosimeters in dose measurements and assigning numbers to each of the quality criteria items, as selected by the human observers. In dose measurements, we need to consider how many repeated measurements are to be carried out and how many decimal numbers are to be recorded. As there is a large uncertainty in low-dose measurements, repeated measurements can improve the accuracy of the dose quantity. We also need to consider operational or other limitations on deciding the number of repeated measurements. For example, too many exposures in a short period may burn the X-ray tube. In assigning numbers to the image quality criteria, we need to consider the number of observers to be used, as there are inter-observer variations. We also need to decide on whether a referencing image or absolute ranking is used and whether observers are reading from printed films or a computer screen for image quality evaluations. All of these operational details can affect the results of measurements.

Finally, data from the measurements should be constantly monitored and assessed during the measurement process to ensure that the data collected are as expected. If not, details of the measurement operation should be reviewed and any incorrect settings or instrument malfunction should be rectified before data collection is continued. For example, we know CTDIv is in the range of 1–100 mGy. If the readings of a dosimeter are significantly outside this range, there could be problems with the ionizing chamber, such as leaking or incorrect settings. In the visual scale grading of image quality example, the researchers should send an initial set of images to the observers for testing. If there is a vast discrepancy between observers in the initial image rankings, then, the researchers should provide the observers with training images for ranking to ensure consistency.

6.3   EXPERIMENTAL DATA COLLECTION STRATEGIES

The most powerful experimental study in clinical investigations is a randomized controlled trial (RCT). The characteristics of an RCT are that it features (1) an intervention or treatment; (2) experimental and control groups; (3) randomized participant selection and group allocation and (4) a statistically significant number of participants. There is a well-defined approach towards data collection in an RCT (Friedman et al., 2015). The RCT approach is considered the true experimental study in other disciplines of social science. Treatment or intervention (manipulation of the dependent variable) differentiates an experimental study from a non-experimental study. Participants in both the experiment (treatment) and control (placebo) groups are required so that data collected from both groups can be contrasted and any effect of the intervention or treatment can be differentiated. Study subjects need to be selected randomly from the population and randomly assigned to the experiment and control groups. The randomized recruitment of participants is to ensure that the participants selected are a true representation of the population, so any findings of the research can be generalized or externally valid. Random subject allocation is closely related to internal validity to ensure any effect on the experimental group is caused by the treatment (intervention). Finally, there must be enough participants to have a statistic-ally significant conclusion. Any bias or non-ideal in this data collection process will have an impact on the results of the trial. The validity of the trial is dependent on how well the treatment is manipulated and the data is collected.

In practice, clinical investigations are often lax versions of an RCT, as the data collection demands of a standard RCT are generally high. For many researchers, it is difficult to meet all the requirements stipulated in an RCT without significant resource backing. The practical strategies in clinical studies are that one follows the standard RCT protocols as closely as possible, considering the data collection limitations of the research environment. For example, we used a non-randomized patient selection strategy and the same patient as their own control in a recent clin-ical study (Zheng et al., 2018). Our approach can be termed a one-group pre-test and post-test in design. Alternatively, we could collect other matching patients' images using general imaging protocols as the control group to the experimental group using our personalized exposure prescription scheme. This could be termed a two-group post-tests only in design. We may also use existing matching patients' images in the PACS database as the control group. This may be termed a time series or historical control in design. These lax versions of the RCT may be termed quasi-experimental studies. Quasi-experimental studies are not as ideal as an RCT but they are valuable contributors in building scientific knowledge. One should remember that scientific evidence is generally accumulated over time and less-powerful clinical investigations can make a big difference to knowledge creation.

Experimental data collection strategies are dependent on available resources and equipment. Researchers must be pragmatic and proactive. In general, the best equipment and data collection strategies, such as those stipulated in an RCT, should be used and followed wherever possible. For example, the standard CT dose phantoms and ionizing chamber dosimeter should be used for CT dose measurements. We sought a loan of the CT dose phantoms and dosimeter from the National Radiation Laboratory of the Australian Radiation Protection and Nuclear Science Agency (ARPANSA) for our measurements. The best available instrument or facility in the world should be used to collect experimental data. For example, we have applied for and been granted access to the Australian Synchrotron for an X-ray tomographic imaging experiment. The Australian Synchrotron is a national research facility of the Australian Nuclear Science and Technology Organization (ANSTO). By using the best instrument, the highest quality of data collected can be assured. In social science, on the other hand, it is believed that the hardest thing in research is to construct an instrument for an abstract concept. The elements of a construct or instrument must not only capture the fundamental characteristics of the concept but its items also have to be quantifiable. It is a good idea to use a proven existing construct or follow existing constructs as closely as possible. For example, we use European image quality criteria (European Commission, 1996) in devising an image quality construct for radiographic chest images: media sternum, parenchyma, bronchus and noise, contrast and abnormality (Zheng, Kim and Yang, 2016). Obviously, other image criteria may be considered but the main image quality factors for a specific clinical task should be included. We may have to construct an instrument ourselves if the preferred instrument is not available or the construct is new.

Data sampling is one of the most important steps in data collection. In the process of participants' recruitment, one must ensure that the data collected from a sample is a true representative of the intended population. Randomization is the key as discussed above. It should also be noted that the methods of data collection and groups being assigned are dependent on your research objectives. For example, if you want to see the difference of interventional effects between male and female, you may divide your sample into male and female subgroups and randomly select subjects from these subgroups for testing. This is called stratified sampling. Various random sampling strategies could be used depending on your research objectives (Bowling, 2014; Friedman et al., 2015). Sample size is another important consideration in data collection. In an RCT, minimum sample size is required for a defined confidence level as stipulated in statistical textbooks (Friedman, 2015). As a rule of thumb for practice, any number less than 30 is generally considered not worthwhile for statistical significance and any number over 1,000 would not make too much of a difference from a statistical test if the sample is truly randomly selected from the population (Bhattacherjee, 2012). Examples for these 'rules of thumb' are that, in our students' experience survey, we generally don't take statistics tests for less than 30 respondents and, in many political polling surveys of voter intentions, one only takes a random sample of 1,000 respondents (Sekarran, 2003). One should also remember that one can still carry out statistical tests for sample size numbers of less than 30, except the errors are expected to be large. Instead of testing for statistical significance, one should consider studies of small numbers as pilot studies, just as the phase I or II studies in randomized controlled trials. As one can see that phase I or II studies are extremely important in RCT, studies involving samples of less than 30 are also important for establishing a case for further studies.

Sampling is also an important data collection step in natural science. The number of data points to be sampled is dependent on the research question. In CT dose measurements, the standard dose measurement points (samplings) are to measure the doses at both the centre and periphery of the CT phantoms. This is because a dose is not uniformly distributed within the body of the phantom – it is higher at the periphery than the body centre. The CT dose index (CTDI) is an average of the measured doses at the centre and periphery of the body. In radiographic imaging, on the other hand, patients' entrance skin doses (ESD) are measured. The patients' absorbed dose in radiographic imaging is generally calculated from the ESD by using Monte Carlo simulations. The standard procedure is to attach a dosimeter to the phantom's surface (the patient's entrance skin). In our studies, we are interested in both the entrance and exit surface doses and the doses at the body centre, so a depth dose profile can be determined. For this reason, the CT dose phantoms are ideal for our purpose in radiographic imaging dose measurements.

Controlling contaminating exogenous or 'nuisance' variables is another important aspect of data collection, particularly when the effect of experimental intervention or a signal is not very strong. For example, assuming we want to remove the gender effect from our comparative study of four groups and there are 20 women among 60 members, we can assign each group with five women so that the effects of gender are distributed across four groups and the confounding effect of gender is cancelled (Cohen, Manion and Morrison, 2007). In our electron density phantom experiment, we were trying to measure the body size effect on CT numbers (Zheng et al., 2020). Because CT numbers are influenced by many factors, the size effects on CT numbers are embedded within other factors including the neighbouring tissue materials. We have to remove all tissue materials from the phantom except for the tissue under study. All the other sample holes within the electron density phantom were filled with water balloons as we don't have extra solid water sample tubes to fill these sample holes. The body size effect on the CT numbers would be indistinguishable from the influence of the neighbouring tissues if the neighbouring tissues were included in the measurements.

Multiple researchers may be involved in data collection, so it is important to ensure consistency in the collection methods. For example, in multi-centre clinical trials, researchers from different organizations may participate in data collection. It is important that a standardized protocol for data collection be developed and agreed at early stage of the study. Everyone should adhere to this pre-defined protocol during the data collection process to ensure consistency and high quality of the data being collected. In the example of image quality evaluations by three experts, the three observers are given the same set of images and the same image quality criteria. If one observer is using a computer screen, one a light box, and the other printed paper to view the image set, clearly, the results would be inconsistent. Consistency is also referred to as internal validity or the degree of confidence that the measured data can be used to establish the causal relationship between variables. In the example of CT dose measurements, confidence in the measured data can be assured by using an ionizing chamber dosimeter that has been calibrated at a national or international standard laboratory.

6.4   NON-EXPERIMENTAL DATA COLLECTION STRATEGIES

Non-experimental data refers to those data that were obtained without manipulating their independent variables. In some cases, it is not possible to manipulate the independent variables for reasons such as ethical considerations. Non-experimental data does not mean that the data cannot be collected from measurements as we have discussed in chapter 5. Non-experimental data are collected from observations (measurements) or existing datasets that have already been collected from measurements for different purposes, such as datasets stored in national organizations, reports of government agencies, and task groups of professional bodies. Secondary data can also be obtained from peer-reviewed scientific journals or textbooks. As discussed before, a systematic review study involves collecting and analysing existing data, either published or unpublished.

One of the most popular non-experimental data collection methods is surveys. The intention of survey studies is not to manipulate independent variables but to seek any causal relationships between the dependent (constructs) and independent variables. As a quantitative methodology, surveys have been used in most fields of study, including sociology, psychology, education, business and medical imaging (Cohnen, Manion and Morrison, 2007; Alewaidat et al, 2018c; Elshami et al., 2019). There are different ways of collecting survey data, such as questionnaires, interviews and observational surveys. For each survey type, there are also sub-type surveys, such as self-administered mail surveys versus group-administered questionnaires. In designing a questionnaire, the choice of the questions' wording, question numbers, order of the questions and the scale for quantization can all have an impact on the results. For example, you can choose 3, 5, 7 or 9 points in a Likert scale or a 100 points scale for your study. One may argue that a 5-point scale is the best for human comparative judgement. The most important part of survey research is ensuring the questions are constructed to test your research question or hypothesis. Our visual grading scale (VGS) study of image quality can be considered a survey study, where human observers are asked to provide responses (image quality scores) to the clinical images based on the image quality criteria. The image ranking can be 3 or 5 points in the Likert scale (Zheng et al., 2015).

The sampling population, sampling method and sample size are all important considerations in survey studies. We may focus on a section of a population, for example, radiographers only or all hospital workers. Sampling can be randomized or nonrandomized. To ensure the survey sample is representative of the intended population, a randomized sampling must be used. For example, in a pre-election survey, a randomized survey of 1,000 voters can be accurate in predicting the results of an election, provided the survey sampling is truly randomized and unbiased. Otherwise, it would provide inaccurate predictions, as we have witnessed in recent US presidential elections. In contrast to traditional paper form survey questionnaires, most contemporary survey data are collected online from the internet, using web-based questionnaires or survey by emails.

In a survey study of patients' awareness and knowledge on the health risks of radiation in CT imaging, we have designed a survey questionnaire and distributed it to six local hospitals (Alewaidat et al., 2018c). The purpose of the study was to assess the current status of radiation awareness among patients – this could lead to an education program being recommended to raise the awareness of radiation protection in the general public. In another study, the levels of radiation protection among health workers were surveyed and personal dose records were reviewed (Elshami et al., 2019). The purpose of the study was to establish if there was any link between the levels of protection and personal dose levels. In this study, the personal dose records were collected from the National Radiation Protection Board. As the survey population was limited to local hospitals, this study was aimed at improving radiation protection practice at a local level. The survey results may not be generalized to a global population, but they can serve as a part of global evidence for generalization.

One of the radiation protection principles in practice is to limit radiation doses to patients. In medical imaging, we have to apply enough exposure (dose) to patients so that the image quality is sufficient for diagnosis. It is inappropriate to set a limit without considering a patient's diagnosis. However, any dose in excess of that required to produce an adequate diagnostic image quality should be avoided (the ALARA principle). A practical way of limiting doses to patients is to establish a dose reference level (DRL) for each of the X-ray imaging protocols, including CT and radiographic imaging (IAEA, 2021). A radiation dose of any imaging protocol exceeding the DRL requires a review and further action may be taken. For a global DRL, a large-scale imaging protocol-based dose survey needs to be carried out across many countries. A localized DRL can also be established by surveying local protocol-based dose data.

These local survey data can also be used in any global surveys. Details of imaging protocols including scan parameters (kVp, mAs, etc.) and other information such as manufacturers' details can be collected from existing PACS systems. A purposely designed survey form, rather than a questionnaire, is used to collect these data. The data collected are not aimed at determining the causal relationship but at establishing an averaged dose level for each of the imaging protocols so that dose reference levels for every imaging protocol can be established.

Existing patients' data in clinical information systems such as a picture archive and communication system (PACS) are often used for retrospective clinical studies. These retrospective data can be used to establish relationships between variables, such as image quality as a function of dose to patients. We collected CT images of various anatomical regions from various local hospitals (Alewaidat et al., 2018a, 2018b). Dose CTDIv, scan parameters as well as other information can be extracted from the images' DICOM header. Human observers are asked to evaluate image quality using a visual grading scale. These collected data can also be used to determine the performances of different CT scanners (models or manufacturers) that a better scanner requires less dose in producing the acceptable image quality for diagnosis. Existing data can be other types or sources, such as the personal dose records from the National Radiation Protection Board (Elshami et al., 2019). Different types of data can be collected and used to establish any relationships between variables, such as questionnaire survey data of radiation protection levels, combined with personal dose records to establish any possible link between personal dose and radiation protection measures.

Accessing data from credible sources or databases is one of the most important strategies in non-experimental data collection. These data sources include peer-reviewed journals, textbooks, research consortia or networks, and national or international organizations including government agencies or bodies. For example, we used data from the National Radiation Protection Board reports in calculating dose correction factors as a function of body size (Hart et al., 2000; Zheng, 2017) and the National Institute of Standards and Technology dataset in determining the Rayleigh scattering cross-section as a function of energy (Berger et al., 2018; Zheng et al., 2020). In general, these data are highly accurate and in the public domain. It is difficult to acquire these data ourselves, given the limited resources and available equipment. Data from peer-reviewed literature can also be used with critical evaluations. In systematic review studies, published or unpublished studies of the same research question are collected and systematically analysed to reach a better conclusion with confidence (Bruce, Pope and Stanistreet, 2018). One may have to contact researchers directly for any unpublished data. Depending on the research question and available data in the public domain, one may have to repeat some measurements to make up for missing information. By repeating published experiments, one may gain further insights or a better understanding of the published data. Some journal reviewers insist on collecting your own data rather than using peer-reviewed experimental results.

Currently, data sharing and open access publishing are 'trendy' in the scientific research community. There are plentiful data sources available, including journals dedicated to dataset publishing, such as *scientific data* from nature research (Scientific data, 2021). Various clinical imaging databases are available in the public domain.

These datasets may be hosted by government agencies or private consortia or joint government and private networks. They offer excellent opportunities for researchers in answering their research questions or testing their hypothesis. For example, the ADNI database for studying Alzheimer's disease is established by the Alzheimer's Disease Neuroimaging Initiative (2021). The ADNI database provides a large number of patients' clinical data and imaging data. Researchers can use this database for many purposes, such as a better understanding and potential treatment of Alzheimer's disease or testing artificial algorithms.

6.5   ENSURING METHODOLOGICAL RELIABILITY AND VALIDITY

Reliability refers to consistency of a measurement and validity refers to the extent to which the scores from a measurement represent the variable they are intended to (Bowling, 2014). In physics, reliability corresponds to precision and validity corresponds to accuracy. The terminologies of internal validity and external validity are also used in scientific research. Internal validity is related to the reliability of the constructs or instrument for the intended variables or elements of the phenomenon. External validity refers to the generalizability of the measurements. Measurements produce two kinds of outcomes: the instrument's indications and knowledge outcome. The instrument outcome is the final state after the measurement is completed while the knowledge outcome is the claims about the values or properties of the object being measured. The goal of scientific research is to create knowledge that is applicable globally. Any research knowledge claims have to be validated with high confidence or within a defined certainty.

To ensure the validity of measured results, one should pay particular attention to the instrument used. In our dose measurement example, we used a dosimeter provided by a manufacturer in our initial experiment but its results were inconsistent with the published standard data. We then sought a loan of CT dose phantoms and an ionizing chamber dosimeter from ARPANSA – the dosimeter had been calibrated at an international standard laboratory (Germany) (Zheng, Nardi and Murray, 2017). In social science research, it is also critical to devise an accurate construct that truly captures the key elements of the abstract concept (Bhattacherjee, 2012). In our visual grading evaluation of image quality, we include clinically relevant criteria and the physical image quality parameters of noise and contrast as part of the image quality items because they are major quality factors for human observers (Zheng et al., 2016). Including trivial or irrelevant factors in the construct may lead to large deviations of measurements from the truth or render the measured results invalid. As stated earlier, one should also monitor the data being collected during the measurement process. Changing the instrument settings and samples are common in data collection. It is important that all settings are correctly set or re-set and all samples are precisely positioned. Any small deviation may result in incorrect or inaccurate results.

Correlating measured results with existing knowledge or literature is another important step in ensuring the validity of measured data. It is expected that measured results will be consistent with existing knowledge and, if not or in doubt, every step in the measuring process should be carefully examined. For example, image quality is expected to be increased if the radiation dose is increased. If our results show the opposite, then, something is going on in the data measurement – for example, the images could be labelled with incorrect doses, the image quality criteria included in the instrument may not be appropriate, or the image quality scores are assigned in the opposite scale direction. In the dose measurement example, we know that the CTDIv is around 20 mGv for abdomen imaging. If the dosimeter gives us an unreasonable value of, say 10 Gray, then something is not right and further investigation is required. It is important that we use existing, proven constructs or regularly calibrated instruments for investigations. If we have to develop our own construct or use an uncalibrated dosimeter, for example, we must test the construct with existing knowledge or calibrate the instrument ourselves against the international standard.

The reliability or precision of a measurement is dependent partly on the measuring instrument and partly on the variables or properties of the phenomenon to be measured. In physics, precision can be determined by repeating the measurements and the standard deviation can then be calculated to determine the precision of the measurements (sometimes we call it error). We repeat each of the CT acquisitions three times to obtain more accurate mean CT values and their standard deviations (Zheng et al., 2020). Standard deviation is also termed uncertainty. The uncertainty gives us an idea of the reliability of the mean values from our measured data. The measured uncertainty is dependent on the measuring instrument, such as the CT scanner and the accuracy of the uncertainty is dependent on the number of repeated measurements. We can repeat our measurements more than three times to gain more accurate CT numbers and their standard deviations. In reality, we need to balance the benefit of gaining the extra statistics with its associated cost. In image quality studies using a visual grading scale, we know that there is a large inter-observer variability, even if the observers are trained experts. A single observer's study is generally not good enough to show the inter-observer's variability. We can ask many observers to evaluate the same set of images using the same visual grading scale to improve the reliability of our measurement. As observer studies of image quality are generally expensive, in practice, we have to balance the number of observers and the study costs.

6.6 CHAPTER SUMMARY

Scientific measurement involves assigning numbers to variables or elements of a phenomenon. There are many aspects or steps in the process of measurement: refining research question(s), precising variable definitions, adjusting or resetting the instrument (construct), determining the scale (unit), testing the operability and monitoring the data being collected. A good research knowledge outcome is guided by scientific intuition and is dependent on a first class (state-of-the-art) instrument and correct execution of the measurement and data collection. Data collection protocols stipulated in randomized controlled trials are the gold standard for any clinical investigations. The key characteristics in RCT data collection are an experimental (treatment) versus control groups, the randomized recruitment of subjects and allocation to groups and a statistically significant number of participants. Many practical data collection protocols less stringent than those of an RCT can be considered quasi-experimental or pilot studies. Quasi-experimental clinical investigations are an important part of building scientific knowledge. The most popular non-experimental data collection approach is the questionnaire survey. The key to survey studies is capturing the key elements of the research question in the construct of the questionnaire items. Imaging information systems including PACS and many publicly available clinical and imaging databases can be valuable non-experimental data sources in answering many research questions. Systematic review studies collect data from published literature or unpublished data. Databases from standard organizations or national and international professional bodies are valuable data sources for theoretical and mathematical analysis in providing answers to research questions. Validity and reliability need be assured to achieve good research outcomes. Reliability refers to consistency of a measurement and validity refers to the extent to which the scores from a measurement represent the variable they are intended to. Scientific knowledge should be globally applicable and knowledge claims have to be validated with high confidence or within a defined certainty.

KEY TERMS

Data sampling: is a statistical technique that is used to analyse patterns and trends in a subset of data in order to represent a larger data set. The sampling determines how much data to collect and how often it should be collected.

Dose reference level: is an indicative dose that is not expected to be exceeded under normal imaging conditions for a given diagnostic procedure.

Imaging information systems: connect and make up a radiology information system, and PACS. The former is used to schedule patient appointments, track examinations, store medical reports and distribute where necessary.

Likert scale: is a scale that is psychometric and commonly involved in research employing questionnaires. It is widely used and can have other types or rating scales attributed to them.

Meta-analysis: is a statistical analysis that combines the results of multiple scientific studies. They are often performed when there are multiple studies addressing the same question.

Sample size: is the act of selecting the number of observations or replicates in a statistical sample. It remains a key feature in empirical work in which inferences about a population are made.

Survey questionnaire: is a word that is used interchangeably that consists of a list of questions aimed at extracting specific data from a particular group of people. Surveys may be conducted by phone, mail or the internet. The latter is often the commonplace.

EXERCISES AND STUDY QUESTIONS

1 Define the four typical measurement scales.
2 Explain the differences between a literature review and systematic review.
3 Explain the characteristics of data collection in randomized controlled trials.

4   Why do we need to control contaminating 'nuisance' variables in data collection?
5   Why is the average inappropriate for numbers in an ordinal scale?
6   Why is the calibration of instruments so important?
7   Why is the sample size (subject numbers) critical?
8   How can the generalizability of knowledge be assured?

REFERENCES

Alewaidat, H., Zheng, X., Khader, Y.S., Theeb, M.A., Alhasan, M.K.M, Rawashdeh, M.A., Al Mousa, D.S. and Alawneh, K.Z.A. (2018a). Assessment of radiation dose and image quality of multidetector computed tomography. *Iranian Journal of Radiology*. 15(3), p. e59554.

Alewaidat, H., Zheng, X., Khader, Y.S., Theeb, M.A., Alhasan, M.K.M., Rawashdeh, M.A.R., Al Mousa, D.S., and Alawneh, K.Z.A. (2018b). Radiation dose and image quality in adult computed tomography scans. *Journal of Medical Imaging and Health Informatics*. 8(2), pp. 223–231.

Alewaidat, H., Zheng, X., Khader, Y., Spuur, K., Abdelrahman, M., Alhasan, M., and Al-Hourani, Z.A. (2018c). Knowledge and awareness of CT radiation dose and risk among patients. *Journal of Diagnostic Medical Sonography*. 34(5), pp. 347–354.

Alzheimer's disease neuroimaging initiative. http://adni.loni.usc.edu/. Accessed on 22-02-2021.

Berger, M.J., Hubbell, J.H., Seltzer, S.M., Chang, J., Coursey, J.S., Sukumar, R., Zuker, D.S., and Olsen, K. XCOM: Photon cross sections database. www.nist.gov/pml/xcom-photon-cross-sections-database. Accessed on 18-11-2018.

Bhattacherjee, A. (2012). *Social Science Research: Principles, Methods, and Practices*. 2nd Edn. Tampa: Open TextBook Publishing.

Bowling, A. (2014). *Research Methods in Health: Investigating Health and Health Services*. 4th Edn. London: Open University Press.

Bruce, N., Pope, D., and Stanistreet, D. (2018). *Quantitative Methods for Health Research: A Practical Interactive Guide to Epidemiology and Statistics*. 2nd Edn. Hoboken: John Wiley & Sons Ltd.

Cohen, L., Manion, L. and Morrison, K. (2007). Research Methods in Education, 6th Edn. London: Routledge Taylor and Francis Group.

Elshami, W., Abuzaid, M., Piersson, A.D., Mira, O., Mohamed AbdelHamid, M., Zheng, X., and Kawooya, M.G. (2019). Occupational dose and radiation protection practice in UAE: A retrospective cross-sectional cohort study (2002–2016). *Radiation Protection Dosimetry*. 187(4), pp. 426–1437

European Commission, 1996. European guidelines on quality criteria for diagnostic radiographic images. Office for Official Publications of European Communities.

Friedman, L.M., Furberg, C.D., DeMets, D.L., Reboussin, D.M., and Granger, C.B. (2015). *Fundamentals of Clinical Trials*. 5th Edn. Heidelberg: Springer.

Hart, D. Wall, B.F., Shrimpton, P.C., and Bungay, D.R. (2000). Reference doses and patient size in paediatric radiology. National Radiological Protection Board Reports (R318). Chilton. UK.

IAEA. Dose reference levels. www.iaea.org/resources/rpop/health-professionals/radiology/diagnostic-reference-levels. Accessed 23-02-2021.

Kothari, C.R. (2004). *Research Methodology: Methods and Techniques*. 2nd Edn. New Age International Publishers.

Scientific data. www.nature.com/sdata/. Accessed on 07-03-2021.

Sekarran, U. (2003). *Research Methods for Business: A Skill-Building Approach*. 4th Edn. New York: John Wiley & Sons, Inc.

Zheng, X. (2017). Patient size based guiding equations for automatic mAs and kVp selections in general medical X-ray projection radiography. *Radiation Protection Dosimetry*. 174(4), pp. 545–550.

Zheng, X.M., Gifford, H.C., Pretorius, P.H., and King, M.A. (2003). An observer study of reconstruction strategies for the detection of solitary pulmonary nodules using hybrid NeoTect SPECT images. *IEEE Nuclear Science Symposium and Medical Imaging Conference Record*. 4, pp. 2690–2694.

Zheng, X., Chiang, H-W., Li, J-H., Chiang, H-J., and Lin, L-H. (2018). Personal exposure prescription method reduces dose in radiography. *Radiologic Technology*. 89(5), pp.435–440.

Zheng, X., Al-Hayek, Y., Cummins, C., Li, X., Nardi, L., Albari, K., Evans, J., Roworth, E., and Seaton, T. (2020). Body size and tube voltage dependent corrections for Hounsfield Unit in medical X-ray computed tomography: Theory and experiments. *Scientific Reports*. 10, p. 15696.

Zheng, X., Kim, T.M., Sook Yang, S., and Kim, Y. (2015). Studies of CT system performances using visual grading scaling: A methodological comparison among visual grading characteristics, ordinal regression and logistic psychometric functions. *International Journal of Computer Assisted Radiology and Surgery*. 10 (Suppl. 1), pp. S5–S6.

Zheng, X., Kim, T.M., and Yang, S. (2016). Optimal kVp in chest computed radiography using visual grading scores: A comparison between visual grading characteristics and ordinal regression analysis. *Proceedings of SPIE (Medical Imaging)*. 9783, pp. 97836A1–97836A8.

Zheng, X., Nardi, L., and Murray, M. (2017). Size effect on dose output in phantoms of X-ray tubes in medical X-ray imaging. *Biomedical Physics and Engineering Express*. 3, p. 065004.

7 Statistical Analysis in Quantitative Research

Xiaoming Zheng

7.1 INTRODUCTION

This chapter considers data analysis in quantitative research. Discrete sample experiments are being carried out in natural science, and small numbers of human subjects are recruited from general populations for experiments in social science. Varied degrees of uncertainties exist in discrete sample studies. Quantitative research is expected to provide a degree of certainty and a level of confidence in the generalization of knowledge claims. Statistical tools are used to analyse measured data from discrete samples. Descriptive statistics are used to describe the characteristics of measured data and any possible relationships among variables. The occurrence frequency or probability density distributions from descriptive statistics can be used for statistical significance tests and integrated as accumulative probability functions for performance tests of various systems. We used the slope of the logistic function between image quality and radiation dose to select the best kVp in CT imaging. Inferential statistics are used to draw conclusions from studies, either by testing relationships drawn from descriptive statistics or theoretical models (hypotheses) for their generalization at a defined level of confidence. The statistical signal detection theory, which originated from the Bayesian theorem, is the basis for both hypothesis testing in randomized controlled trials and receiver operating characteristics (ROC) studies in radiology, as well as many practical statistical tests. A generalized linear regression model can be used to establish causal relationships among multiple variables of measured data in multiple measurement scales. We used a generalized linear model for ordinal regression in determining the best kVp for chest X-ray imaging.

7.2 WHY DO WE NEED STATISTICS?

We live in an uncertain world and make decisions every day based on existing knowledge with various degrees of uncertainty. We would like to have knowledge about everything and understand exactly how things work so that we can make favourable, informed decisions. Unfortunately, this is not the case. There are many questions to be answered and so much unknown information to be discovered. That is why

DOI: 10.1201/9780367559311-7

research is so important. We wish research could provide us with precise knowledge so that we can be assured in our everyday decision-making. In reality, this is not possible. Uncertainty is a part of nature and our lives. Uncertainty or variability of a research outcome can be large or small but uncertainty is always there. As uncertainty is a part of nature, we would like at least to know the extent to which the knowledge is applicable or to be certain about the uncertainty. Statistical analysis can provide us with the needed certainties and levels of confidence from our research.

In classical mechanics, the variability of measurements is relatively small or at least acceptable within certain expectations. Statistics is thus not often used in some studies of classical mechanics (Hill and Zheng, 1996). In quantum physics, however, the uncertainty of a particle's position is extremely large or unpredictable based on conventional expectations. The entire study of quantum mechanics is based on statistics or probability density functions (Zheng and Smith, 1991). In studies of radiation effects on human tissues, the predictions range from deterministic at high doses to stochastic at low radiation doses. At low doses, there is a large uncertainty in measuring the doses (Zheng, 2016a), let alone the tissue responses to the low dose radiations. It appears that the best statistical tools are unable to reach a conclusion as far as the tissue response to the low-dose radiation is concerned (ICRP, 2007). The international community has to extrapolate the tissue responses from high doses, such as in radiotherapy, and deduce it from epidemiologic studies (ibid). The linear non-threshold model for the low-dose regime adopted by the United Nations Scientific Committee for Radiation Protection remains a controversial question in the scientific community. In social science or psychology, there is a (reasonably) large uncertainty in measuring human subjects' behaviours. Statistical analysis of social or psychological measurements is necessary to provide a level of certainty on the uncertainties of the knowledge generated by research and a level of confidence in the translations of research findings into a general population. The generalization of research findings in natural science is largely via repeated measurements by independent researchers and laboratories. In contrast, large-scale experiments on human subjects are generally uneasy, if not impossible. A sample of a small number of human subjects is often drawn from a population for an experiment. The important question is how reliably can the experimental results from a small sample of human subjects be generalized to a general population? Statistics is the best tool to answer this question.

7.3   DESCRIPTIVE STATISTICS

Descriptive statistics, as the name suggests, describe the characteristics of the measured data. The term refers to various techniques in the summarizing, displaying and statistical fitting of possible relationships from measured data. In our CT experiments, we repeat CT image acquisitions three times and average CT numbers from eight central slices of the electron density phantom (Zheng et al., 2020). The averaged CT values and their standard deviations are the basic characteristics of the measured data from the simplest statistics. We take the averaged CT numbers because CT numbers are inherently noisy (uncertain), due to the sources such as photon number fluctuations, photon beam filtrations, beam hardening and image-reconstruction algorithms. The standard deviation tells us the variation or uncertainty of the measured CT values that we would like to know. Digital CT images' values are in Hounsfield units. We can display these Hounsfield numbers in a histogram that shows the occurrence or frequency distribution of these CT numbers within the image. In image segmentation, we can use the histogram of an image to set thresholds for the separation of different anatomical regions based on modes within the histogram. In our serum caffeine level study (Zheng and Williams, 2002), we present the numbers of patients with certain serum caffeine levels in a histogram to show the caffeine level distributions among patients. It gives us a visual summary of the collected data. Much characteristic information can be extracted from a histogram distribution of the measured data by simple statistical analysis. Apart from the above mean values and standard deviation, the skewness and kurtosis can also be extracted from the histogram of measured data. Skewness is a measure of symmetry or asymmetry. The distribution of a dataset is symmetric if it looks the same to the left and right of the centre point. Kurtosis is a measure of whether the data are heavy-tailed or light-tailed relative to a normal distribution. The occurrence frequency distribution (histogram) of measured data can be converted to a probability distribution if we normalize the occurrence frequencies by the total number of the events (total pixels in an image). These measured probability distributions can be used for further statistical tests or analysis. Different mean values, standard deviations, shapes and tails of these measured probability distributions will influence the accuracy of statistical tests. An integration of the probability or frequency distribution will produce a sigmoid curve or accumulative probability function. The sigmoid function is a typical optical density function (H&D curve) in radiography (Bonciu, Rezaee and Edwards, 2006), typical treatment control function in radiotherapy (Joiner and van der Kogel, 2009) and typical psychometric function in psychology (Gescheider, 1997).

In establishing a local dose reference level (LDRL) for an imaging protocol, the number of patients versus received doses are displayed in a histogram and a dose at 75% of all patient doses is set as the dose reference level for the specific imaging protocol. For national or international dose reference levels (NDRLs), one can display the number of hospitals (facilities) versus LDRL and an LDRL at 75% of all facilities surveyed can be set as the NDRL for that specific imaging protocol (Lee et al., 2020). The distributions of the number of patients versus received doses or the number of facilities (hospitals) versus LDRLs can be integrated as accumulated percentage of patients (facilities) versus received doses (LDRLs). Again, the DRL (NDRL) is set at a dose value corresponding to an accumulated 75% of all patients surveyed. The display of accumulated percentage number of patients versus received doses is the same as the histogram display of patient numbers (frequency) versus received doses, except that the former is accumulated patient numbers (in percentage or normalized) versus the received doses. The accumulated frequency distribution is more intuitive as its vertical axis is in a percentage scale, which has a corresponding value of 75% as the threshold. The 75% is a consensus value that is acceptable in many clinical decisions. The slope at 50% of accumulative frequency distributions may be used as an index for measuring the spread of dose distributions between different imaging protocols.

In psychophysics studies of human perception, including the perception of medical images, researchers apply a physical stimulus to human subjects and measure their responses (Gedcheider, 1997). To determine a threshold strength of sound for human perception, psychophysicists produce different sounds with varied intensities and ask human subjects to confirm if they heard a sound or not. The measured data can be plotted as the frequency of a human subject's responses to 'yes' versus sound strengths. This plot is called a psychometric function and the sound strength for a 50% correct response is taken as the threshold strength. The psychometric function is an accumulated probability function and its differentiation is the frequency (density) distribution as discussed earlier. Several typical psychometric functions have been demonstrated in various psychophysics studies, such as logit, logistic, accumulated normal, and Weibull functions (Strasburger, 2001). Taking the accumulated normal function as an example, its differentiation is a normal distribution. The slope of the accumulated normal function is an indication of the standard deviation of the normal distribution, which is an important characteristic of the measured data. The slope of a psychometric function can be used to measure the performances of human subjects or instruments (Zheng et al., 2014). In radiography, the slope of the optical density function (H&D curve) is a performance index for the radiographic imaging system (Bonciu and Rezaee, 2006).

In medical imaging, we produce images with varied image quality (varied doses) and ask human observers (radiologists) to determine (response) if the image is acceptable for diagnosis or not. This is just one of the psychophysics studies like the perception of sound discussed earlier. Using a five-point Likert scale is equivalent to asking human subjects for more detailed responses: 1, definitely unacceptable; 2, below acceptable; 3, just acceptable, 4, above acceptable and 5, definitely acceptable. A plot of the human observers' image quality responses (rankings) versus the doses linked to the images is a psychometric function (Zheng et al., 2015). Various psychometric functions can be produced by ranking images under different conditions such as different kVps or image reconstruction algorithms of CT images. The slopes of these psychometric functions can be used to measure the performances of imaging techniques (comparing different kVps) or reconstruction algorithms (comparing FBP with iterative reconstructions) or human observers. The differentiation of the psychometric function of diagnostic image quality versus radiation dose led to a general equation for optimal selections of scan parameters, kVp and mAs, in X-ray imaging including CT and radiographic imaging (Zheng, 2016b; Zheng, 2017b). For the first time, the two imaging modalities of CT and radiographic imaging became united under one operational equation (Zheng, 2017b; Zheng, 2018).

The above links between frequency distribution functions and psychometric (sigmoid) functions show the importance of examining the measured data using descriptive statistics. Frequency distribution and probability distribution are interchangeable depending on the research questions. Not only can these measured frequency distributions be converted to psychometric functions (the slopes of which are used as a performance index) but also the probability distributions of measured control (normal, background) and experimental (treatment, signal) groups can also be used for statistical significance tests. Different distribution characteristics of the measured data, such as the mean and standard deviation, skewness and kurtosis, will lead to different psychometric functions for performance tests and different results for statistical significance tests because different shapes and tails will result in different probability overlaps (i.e., types I and II errors) between signal (treatment) and background (control) distributions.

Descriptive statistics are often being used to establish the best fit mathematical functions or relationships between variables for measured data. For example, to establish the relationship between image quality and dose, we can use Microsoft Excel to plot the measured data of image quality versus dose (Zheng, 2016b). We then test for a few probable relationship functions and calculate their correlation coefficient, r. If $r=0$, the data does not fit for the selected function, and if $r=1$, the measured data is a perfect match for the selected function. Here, r is calculated based on the differences between the measured data and the assumed mathematical function. Microsoft Excel provides a few popular functions such as linear, logarithmic, exponential, polynomial or power functions and correlation coefficients with the measured data, r, can be calculated for each of these functions. A function with the highest r can be selected as the best fit in describing the relationship of the measured data. In determining the best function for the measured data, no attempt has been made to generalize the function to a general population. This is often the case in natural science research because generalization in natural science is often through validation from independent researchers and independent laboratories. To determine if the best relationship function is generalizable or statistically significant, inferential statistics or a statistical test is required. The correlation coefficient r is only one of the parameters in a statistical significance test. We seldom carry out statistical tests for generalizability in natural science research but we consider a fitting function with $r>0.95$ as a good fit. In the field of psychology, it is suggested that a correlation coefficient of $r\sim0.8$ is strong, $r\sim0.5$ is medium and $r\sim0.2$ is considered weak for statistical power tests (Price, Jhangiani and Chiang, 2015). The expectation of $r>0.95$ in natural science research is well above the $r\sim0.80$ level, so the generalizability appears to be assured or is statistically significant.

The curve fittings of relationships between variables may be considered as nonparametric statistics where no function is pre-assumed. We estimate the correlation coefficients, r, on various likely functions, so that the highest r is selected as the best function for the measured data. If we have reasons to believe that our measured data follow a specific distribution function (or accumulative function) such as a normal distribution, we can fit the measured data to the assumed distribution function. The parameters for the assumed distribution function can be estimated using statistical analysis on the measured data, such as the mean value and standard deviation for a normal distribution. This analysis is termed parametric statistics. For example, imagine we have collected 128 T1-weighted MRI images of Alzheimer's patients and would like to determine the mean value and standard deviation of patients' hippocampus volume. We can calculate the patients' hippocampus volumes using freely available software and use descriptive statistics in the SPSS package to determine the mean value and standard deviation of the hippocampus volumes, assuming a normal distribution. The histogram of the hippocampus volumes or volume occurrence frequencies can be compared with the expected frequencies from a normal distribution. It can pick up any missing data by comparing the measured data with the expected normal distribution.

The probability distributions constructed by measured data using a small number of subjects may be inaccurate – their accuracy can be improved by adding more subjects into the statistics. A systemic review and meta-analysis are used to improve the statistics by combining a number of studies involving small subject numbers (Bruce, Pope and Stanistreet, 2018). Meta-analysis uses each of the individual studies as a block in the combined statistical analysis. This is equivalent to the national DRL that uses local hospitals' (facilities') DRLs as blocks in the construction of the NDRLs (Lee et al., 2020). The process of establishing accurate probability (frequency) distributions of variables can be considered as knowledge building. Initial probability distributions may be constructed by a small number of subjects and can be improved over time by gradually adding more subjects. Radiologists make diagnostic decisions based on their knowledge, which is usually gained gradually from training in reading diagnostic images for clinical tasks. Radiologists' training is equivalent to building probability density maps in their mind (brain) and their knowledge (probability distribution) improving with experience. In artificial intelligence or an artificial neural network (Zheng et al., 2004), the training data are used to establish the weighting (probability) functions for each of the input nodes or dependent variables. There is an activation function that links the input nodes to the output nodes in the next layer of the network (ibid). The activation function for a node is generally a sigmoid function such as a logistic, logit, accumulative normal or step function. These activation functions are similar to those psychometric functions in describing our image quality and dose relationships (Zheng et al., 2014;2015;2016). The slopes of these activation (psychometric) functions are the weightings (measures) of the nodes (systems). The summation of these weightings triggers an activation (decision) for output to the next layers of the artificial neural network (Zheng et al., 2004).

7.4   INFERENTIAL STATISTICS

Inferential statistics are the statistical tools used to draw conclusions from measured data. We use descriptive statistics to describe the characteristics of measured data or suggest a best relationship function for the measured data. No attempt is made to generalize the results to a general population. To make research findings conclusive, a statistical test is required, particularly for results from samples with small numbers drawn from large populations. Research can be inductive or deductive or both, depending on the question. Deductive research is trying to test a theory or model (hypothesis test). Inductive research is trying to establish a theory or mathematical relationships (laws) between variables from the measured data, which are expected to be further tested. In the image quality and dose optimization example, we derived equations for optimal selections of scan parameters kVp and mAs given a patient's body thickness (Zheng, 2016b; Zheng, 2017a). These equations have been further tested, such as in the clinical trial of chest imaging using a c-arm radiographic imaging system (Zheng et al., 2018). As stated in chapter 6, any knowledge claims from scientific research must be valid both internally and externally. The external validity in natural science is expected to be validated by independent researchers and the expectation of uncertainty is relatively small – the correlation coefficient r is expected to be larger than 0.95. In social science, however, repeat or alternative experiments on human subjects are generally difficult – experiments on human subjects are generally limited by small numbers of subjects drawn from large populations. Their external validity or generalizability is better tested by inferential statistics than by independent human experiments. Statistical testing aims to provide an assurance of the validity of the study in the absence of independent experiments. Of course, validations by independent experiments on human subjects would be better but they are difficult to organize. Discrete sampled experiments in natural science are frequently carried out. Because statistical significance tests are not frequently carried out, natural scientists would not consider an $r\sim0.8$ as a strong correlation. In contrast, in psychology, $r\sim0.8$ is considered strong if one is going to carry out a statistical significance test (Price, Jhangiani and Chiang, 2015). To draw a conclusion, it is recommended that a statistical test be carried out on all results from discrete sample experiments both for natural and social sciences.

To test if a correlation is statistically significant or generalizable, we can calculate a value called t, that takes into account the r-value calculated from the measured data and the sample number, n (Kothari, 2004). The resulting t-value can be compared with values in a t table. The t table lists t values under different degrees of freedom and levels of confidence. If the calculated t value is larger than the value in the table under the defined significance level (say 5%) and the sample's degrees of freedom, the correlation is considered statistically significant or generalizable to the general population (ibid). In the descriptive statistics discussion, we stated that measured data can be displayed as a histogram or frequency (probability) distribution. We may ask if the measured data follows a normal distribution or not and if yes, if the measured data as a normal distribution can be generalized to the general population. We can carry out a χ^2 test (Kothari, 2004), which is calculated as the ratio of the standard deviation and the mean value of the measured data multiplied by the degree of freedom ($n-1$) of the sample. This χ^2 value is then compared with the χ^2 table, where the values are listed under various significance levels and degrees of freedom for a normal distribution. If the calculated χ^2 value is larger than the value in the table under the defined significance level (say 5%) and the sample's degrees of freedom, the normal distribution is rejected or the measured data have a statistically different distribution from the normal distribution in the general population. One can see that there are three elements in this statistical significance test: (1) sample number; (2) assumed distribution and (3) significance level. The sample number (size) n is an important factor in the statistical significance test. The sample number will have a large impact on the results to be generalized if the number is small. The significance level is the risk one is prepared to take for the results to be generalized. The smaller the percentage level, the harder to achieve the defined level of statistical significance. There are assumed distributions for the t or χ^2 values to be tabled under various significance levels and degrees of freedom (parametric). The same concept applies to the statistical significance tests of many other correlations, curve fittings or distributions from the measured data.

In clinical trials, we often use the terminology of hypothesis test (Friedman et al., 2015). It should be noted that hypothesis test is a general term and most research questions can be considered as hypothesis tests. In an RCT, we are testing two hypotheses: (1) there is no effect (null hypothesis) H_0 and (2) there is a difference (the alternative) H_1. The purpose of this test is to see whether or not the new drug, treatment, device or protocol can be applied to the general population. The test results will be used by policymakers to approve or disapprove its usage by the general population. One can understand that patients' safety is the absolute priority and must be at the forefront of any tests of the effectiveness of drugs or devices. The hypothesis test is equivalent to saying that there is no effect (no difference) unless proven beyond doubt. In other words, we need to be sure that the proven effectiveness or the probability of the effectiveness is very high for the drug or device to be used in the general population. We set a small probability of a 5% false-positive fraction or type I error $\alpha = 0.05$, which is termed the confidence level. In other words, we accept only a 5% risk of negative (normal) being identified as positive. For the RCT studies discussed in Chapter 6, we have two (experimental and control) human subjects' groups and both the recruitment and group assignment of human subjects are randomized. Once the data are collected, we can calculate the true-positive and false-positive (type I error, α) fractions and true-negative and false-negative (type II error, β) fractions and mean difference (μ) between the two groups. If $\alpha < 0.05$, we say that the drug is effective (H_0 is rejected) with a confidence α, or it is statistically significant. By saying this, we are taking a risk of a 5% possibility the drug is not effective.

There are two drug (treatment) effectiveness distributions of experimental and control groups in the above hypothesis test. These two distributions are constructed by the measured data. The mean drug effect (μ) is the mean difference between the two distributions. We can assume normal distributions of drug effectiveness for both experiment and control groups, as the data were collected from randomized subjects' recruitment and groups' assignment. The accuracy of the normal distribution assumption will depend on the randomness of the subjects' recruitment and groups' assignment in data collection. The measured effectiveness distributions may have different shapes or tails to the normal distribution, which will affect the accuracy of the type I and type II error calculations. Another factor that will affect the accuracy is the sample size or number of subjects who participated in the trial, particularly if the number of participants is small because the recruitment of human subjects is generally not easy. The estimation of the two drug effectiveness distributions is dependent on the number of subjects. The accuracies of type I error or confidence level α, type II error β and the mean difference μ are all dependent on the sample sizes (numbers). The statistical power is defined as the probability of correctly rejecting the null hypothesis, H_0, or ($1-\beta$) (Friedman et al., 2015). It quantifies the potential of the study to find the true differences of various values μ. Since β is dependent on α, μ and the sample size, the statistical power is also dependent on these parameters. In practice, we would like to have a statistical power of a minimum of 0.80, preferably 0.90 or 0.95 (ibid). In other words, we would like to have an 80%, a 90% or 95% chance of finding a statistical difference between the experiment and control groups. In setting the confidence level at $\alpha = 0.05$, we are prepared for a 5% risk of incorrectly identifying the drug as effective while, in fact, it has no effect. We can set more strict levels such as 2.5% or 1% depending on the risk one is prepared to take. The statistical power will be higher but demand for other parameters such as sample size and mean difference will be larger.

In radiology, the gold standard methodology for the assessment of clinical studies is ROC studies (Zheng et al., 2003; Mets, 2006). ROC studies can be used to assess the performances of imaging systems, imaging protocols, software such as iterative image reconstruction, or the performance of radiologists themselves. A ROC study is based on clinical outcomes, i.e., any technology or clinical innovation must demonstrate improved performance for patients' diagnosis and management. In a typical ROC study, such as in the performance assessment of image reconstruction algorithms between filtered back-projection and the iterative reconstruction algorithms for the detection of solitary pulmonary nodules (Zheng et al., 2003), human observers were asked to assess a total of 324 images, of which half (162) were normal and half (162) were abnormal. These images were reconstructed by both the iterative reconstruction algorithm with varied iteration as well as the filtered back-projection algorithm. Human observers were asked to decide if the image was normal or a tumour was present. Human observers' decisions used a six-point scale, corresponding to different decision thresholds. For each of the reconstruction algorithms and decision thresholds, the observers' true-positive fraction (TPF), false-positive fraction (FPF, type I error, α), true-negative fraction (TNF) and false-negative fraction (FNF, type II error, β) were calculated. These results were plotted in a 2D diagram where the y-axis was the TPF and the x-axis was 1-TNF. By linking (fitting) the data points of one image reconstruction technique with different decision thresholds, we obtained a ROC curve. The area under the ROC curve, Az, is the performance index to be used to compare different reconstruction algorithms.

In the ROC studies above, we used an equal number of images depicting normal and diseased patients. Unlike RCT studies, the numbers for normal and diseased patients in ROC studies can be different, such as in lung or breast screening studies where the normal patients' numbers are much larger than the diseased patients. Similar to RCT studies, there is a normal group and a diseased group, and there are normal and diseased probability distributions for these groups. In ROC studies, the ROC curve is produced by varying the observer's decision thresholds, which is equivalent to scanning through the two probability distributions. These two probability distributions generally overlap, and this overlap is the source of type I (α) and type II (β) errors or false-positive and false-negative fractions. Unlike hypothesis tests in which the type I error (α) is a pre-set confidence level, the type I and type II errors in ROC studies are existing facts, and the ROC curve reveals these facts (including the type I and type II errors). By scanning through the two probability distributions, the mean difference (μ) between the two distributions and the standard deviations of these two distributions can be estimated. A detectability index d' is often used to measure the performance of a clinical system where d' is the ratio of the mean difference (μ) and the joint standard deviation of the two distributions (Macmillan and Creelman, 2004). Not surprisingly, the detectability index is equivalent to the area under the ROC curve, Az.

One can see from the above discussions, the fundamental statistics for hypothesis tests and ROC studies are the same, in which two probability distributions are measured and used for these tests. The two probability distributions of signal (treatment, diseased) and noise (background, normal, control) are the foundation of statistical signal detection theory (Wickens, 2002). The signal detection theory can be considered an expression of the Bayesian theorem (ibid). In a ROC study, the two distributions are measured (sampled) by varying the decision thresholds, while in hypothesis tests in RCT studies, the two distributions are measured from the (sampled) control and treatment groups. In ROC studies, we can estimate a ROC curve without varying the decision thresholds if normal distributions for both normal and diseased can be assumed under the condition of randomized patient recruitment and group assignment (this requirement is not enforced in ROC studies). This is because the two probability distributions can be determined by the TPF, FPF, TNF and FNF at a single decision point under the normal distribution assumption. In a ROC study, the mean difference between the signal and background is given (existing facts), while the mean difference of the drug effect in an RCT between the experiment and control groups is to be established as a part of the statistical significance test. The type I error α can be calculated ($\alpha = 1$-TPF) in ROC studies while α in a hypothesis test is a given (pre-set confidence level). Although the statistical tools are the same for both hypothesis tests and the ROC studies, the objectives of these two studies are different. The hypothesis test is aimed at ensuring the risk of taking a drug (treatment) is small. The ROC study is aimed at determining which technology, such as the best kVp in X-ray CT or radiographic imaging, is better at revealing the true status of a disease.

One can see that presenting measured data using descriptive statistics such as frequency distribution (histogram) or probability distribution can be considered the first step in drawing a conclusion from the inferential statistics (hypothesis test, ROC study). Different (frequency, probability) distribution functions or different mean values, standard deviations, shapes and tails of a probability distribution will have different impacts on the accuracies of the conclusions. One can assume some typical probability distributions, such as a normal distribution, use the measured data to estimate the parameters of the assumed distribution (parametric statistics) then proceed to carry out the tests. One can also construct the probability distributions directly from the measured data (non-parametric statistics) and proceed to carry out the test. For example, let's assume that the hippocampus volume can be used to decide if a patient has Alzheimer's disease (AD) and that we have the measured hippocampus volume distributions both for normal controls and AD patients. We can use these two distributions to construct a likelihood observer to test if a patient has AD or not, given the patient's hippocampus volume. The likelihood is based on signal detection theory and can be considered an application of the Bayesian theorem (Wickens, 2002).

Many of the popular statistical tests (Kothari, 2004) can be interpreted in the same way as RCT and ROC studies. For example, let's assume we are using the Wilcoxon matched-pair test to determine if there is any difference between two brands of the same product (ibid). We can ask customers, say $n = 30$, to rank them on a 100-point scale. We have 30 paired ranking values for the two brands. The procedure in the Wilcoxon test is as follows: (1) calculate the differences of all pairs (remove zero difference pairs and n is reduced by the number of zero pairs); (2) use the absolute ranking (value) differences (the smallest pair is 1, use the averaged number for equal difference pairs); (3) calculate the test statistic W and (4) compare the calculated W with the W table under a specific confidence level, say $\alpha = 0.05$. If the calculated W is larger than the tabled value, then the H_0 hypothesis is rejected or there is a statistically significant difference between the two brands. In this test, we assumed that there is no difference between the two brands, H_0. It means that the signed-ranks should be symmetrically distributed around zero with an n specific variance. For the pair numbers $n > 30$, this symmetrical distribution would be very close to a normal distribution. If the distribution of the measured ranks (H_1) is shifted from zero (H_0 distribution), there is a difference between the measured (H_1) and assumed distribution (H_0) with an overlap between the H_0 and H_1 distributions. At $\alpha = 0.05$, the shift of the H_1 distribution from the H_0 distribution has to be large enough so that there is only 5% of the measured distribution H_1 overlapping with the H_0 distribution. Otherwise, we would keep the H_0 hypothesis even though there is a shift of the measured H_1 distribution from the assumed H_0 distribution, i.e., the mean difference, $\mu \neq 0$. The confidence level has an impact on the decision of whether we should reject H_0 or not.

In descriptive statistics, we discussed the curve fittings for measured data. For example, we like to see if the measured data fit a linear function or not by calculating the correlation coefficient r. This curve fitting process is conventionally termed linear regression, where the difference between the measured data and the expected (linear) function is calculated and the correlation coefficient r, the goodness of fit, is calculated. One can go on to test its statistical significance for generalization. For data in ratio or interval scales, the establishment of the causal relationship appears straightforward using conventional linear regression. For nominal or ordinal data types, however, the conventional curve fitting process may not be applicable because the values in ordinal or categorical scales are nominal numbers – ordinal numbers are meaningful in their order only. The values corresponding to an ordinal number are in some kind of distribution and their mean value does not necessarily equal the ordinal number. Nominal numbers are for classification only. To determine the causal relationships between dependent variables and independent variables for ordinal and nominal numbers, a generalized linear regression model has been developed (DeCarlo, 1998). The term 'regression' is similar to the curve fittings discussed but a link function (assumed accumulated probability function such as logit, logistic and accumulated normal) is used to fit the measured values. As in conventional linear regression, the dependent variable Y is expressed as being linearly proportional to the dependent variable X with a linear coefficient, a, and intercept, b, where a is the slope of the line if it is plotted on a graph as a conventional linear function. Unlike in conventional linear regression, the measured variables of ordinal or categorical scales are in some kind of distribution and we can nominate a distribution function or a link function (accumulated probability distribution function) for them. We have seen that the slopes of the accumulated distribution function or sigmoid functions are performance measures (indexes) (Zheng et al., 2014). For example, in determining the optimal kVp in CT imaging, we used the slopes of the psychometric function (image quality versus radiation doses) where the best kVp has the highest slope of the psychometric function (Zheng et al., 2015). The slopes or linear coefficients of the independent variables X in the generalized linear model are also the 'performance' measures, where a larger slope means that the dependent variable Y is dependent more on this particular independent variable, either in positive or negative ways. The generalized linear regression model can handle multiple independent variables and dependent variables in multiple measurement scales. 'Dummy' variables are used for categorical variables in SPSS software. The resulting coefficients of the independent variables from the regression indicate the response rates (positive or negative) of the particular variables, i.e., a larger coefficient of an independent variable suggests that this independent variable carries more weight than other variables to the response of the dependent variable (Zheng, Kim and Yang, 2016). The generalized linear regression model can be used in many fields of science, including business and education (Bhattacherjee, 2012).

In our visual grading scale (VGS) studies of image quality, both image quality and image quality criteria are in ordinal scales. Image quality is the dependent variable and image quality criteria items are the independent (multiple) variables. We can use the generalized linear regression model to establish the causal relationships by setting image quality as the dependent variable and image quality criteria items as the independent variables. In our study (Zheng, Kim and Yang, 2016), we were interested in the optimal kVp or the impact of various kVps on image quality. We set various kVps as the independent variables instead and the best kVp is determined by comparing the coefficients (slopes) of the independent variables in the regression model (locations in the SPSS software) (ibid). The statistical tests or the confidence levels are part of the regression analysis based on the number of data samples (degree of freedom) and the link function (assumed distribution function).

7.5 CHAPTER SUMMARY

Uncertainty is a part of nature and our lives. It can be large or small but it is always there. Scientific knowledge must be validated and generalizable in the general population. Quantitative research attempts to provide knowledge with a degree of certainty. Discrete sample experiments are carried out in natural science, and small numbers of human subjects are recruited from general populations for experiments in social science. Statistical tools are used to analyse experimental data from discrete samples. Descriptive statistics are used to describe the characteristics of the sampled data and attempt to establish any relationships between variables so that theoretical models or frameworks may be constructed for further testing. The occurrence frequency or probability distributions from descriptive statistics can be used for further statistical tests or performance tests of different systems if they are integrated into accumulative probability functions. Inferential statistics are used to draw conclusions from studies, either by testing relationships drawn from the descriptive statistics or testing the theoretical models (hypotheses) for generalizability with a level of confidence. The statistical signal detection theory is the basis for both the hypothesis test in randomized controlled trials and the receiver operating characteristic studies in radiology as well as many of the practical statistical tests. A generalized linear regression model can be used to establish causal relationships among multiple variables of measured data in multiple measurement scales.

KEY TERMS

Accumulative probability function: refers to the probability that the value of a random variable falls within a specific range.

Area under the ROC curve: is a graphical tool that depicts the diagnostic ability of a binary classifier as its threshold is varied.

Confidence level: or interval is a type of estimate computed from the statistics of the observed data. It gives a range of values for an unknown parameter.

Correlation coefficient: is a statistical measure of the strength of the relationship between the variance between two variables, which range between -1.0 and 1.0.

Curve fitting: is a process of constructing a curve or mathematical function that has the best fit to a series of data points.

Descriptive statistics: is the statistical summary statistic that quantitatively describes features of collected information. It seeks to sort and analyse these statistics for presentation.

Generalizability: is the term used to measure how useful research data is to a broader group of people or situations.

Generalized linear regression model: is a term that refers to the conventional linear regression model for continuous response variables that are given continuous or categorical predictors.

Histogram: is a graphical representation of data using bars of differing heights. It is used to demonstrate the distribution of numerical data.

Inferential statistics: is a field of statistics using during data analysis which seeks to infer outcomes to underlying distribution of probability. Inferential statistics seeks to infer properties onto a larger population.

Probability distribution: falls into probability theory and statistics that gives probabilities of occurrence of different possible outcomes for an experiment. It mathematically describes random phenomena in terms of their sample spacing.

Psychometric function: is an inferential model applied in the detection and discrimination tasks and seeks to identify relationships between features such as physical stimulus.

Sigmoid function: is a mathematical function that has a characteristic 'S' shaped curve and is commonly used as a logistic function, as observed in radiography.

Signal detection theory: offers a means to measure and differentiate between patterns of information, such as the differences between signal and noise in digital images.

EXERCISES AND STUDY QUESTIONS

1   What is a probability density distribution function? How do you calculate a probability density distribution's mean, standard deviation, skewness and kurtosis?

2   What is a hypothesis test? Why do we need hypothesis tests?

3   What is a ROC study in radiology? How do you determine a radiologist's performance using a ROC study?

4   What is the confidence level? How is the confidence level defined in the framework of signal detection theory?

5   What is statistical power? How would you determine statistical power in a randomized controlled trial?

6   What are sensitivity, specificity, type I errors and type II errors?

7   What is the relationship between a probability distribution and an accumulative probability function?

8   Explain how to carry out a generalized linear regression analysis in determining the causal relationships among variables of a phenomenon.

REFERENCES

Bhattacherjee, A. (2012) *Social Science Research: Principles, Methods, and Practices*. 2nd Edn. Tampa: OpenTextBook Publishing.

Bonciu, C., Rezaee, M.R. and Edwards, W. (2006) Enhanced visualization methods for computed radiography images. *Journal of Digital Imaging*. 19(2), pp. 187–196.

Bruce, N., Pope, D. and Stanistreet, D. (2018) *Quantitative Methods for Health Research: A Practical Interactive Guide to Epidemiology and Statistics*. 2nd Edn. Hoboken: John Wiley & Sons Ltd.

DeCarlo, L.T. (1998) Signal detection theory and generalized linear model. *Psychological Methods*. 3(2), pp. 186–205.

Friedman, L.M., Furberg, C.D., DeMets, D.L., Reboussin, D.M. and Granger, C.B. (2015) *Fundamentals of Clinical Trials*. 5th Edn. Heidelberg: Springer.

Gescheider, G.A. (1997) *Psychophysics: The Fundamentals*. 3rd Edn. London: Lawrence Erlbaum Associates Publishers.

Hill, J.M. and Zheng, X.M. (1996). Dilatant double shearing theory applied to granular chute flow. *Acta Mechanica*. 118, pp. 97–108.

ICRP. Publication 103. (2007). The 2007 recommendations of the international commission on radiological protection. *Ann ICRP*. 37.

Joiner, M. and van der Kogel, A. (Eds.). 2009. *Basic Clinical Radiobiology*. Published in Great Britain by Holder Arnold, a Hachette UK company.

Kothari, C.R. 2004. *Research Methodology: Methods and Techniques*. 2nd Edn. New Delhi: New Age International Publishers.

Lee, K.L., Beveridge, T., Sanagou, M. and Thomas, P. (2020). Updated Australian diagnostic reference levels for adult CT. *Journal of Medical Radiation Sciences*. 67, pp. 5–15.

Macmillan, N.A. and Creelman, C.D. (2004). *Detection Theory: A User's Guide*. Hoboken: Taylor and Francis.

Mets, C.E. (2006). Receiver operating characteristic analysis: A tool for quantitative evaluation of observer performance and imaging systems. *Journal of the American College of Radiology*. 3, pp. 413–422.

Price, P.C., Jhangiani, R.S. and Chiang, I-C. A. (2015). *Research Methods in Psychology*. 2nd Canadian Edn. Fresno: BCcampus Publisher.

Strasburger, H. (2001) Converting between measures of slope of psychometric function. *Perception & Psychophysics*. 63(8), pp. 1348–1355.

Wickens, T.D. (2002). *Elementary Signal Detection Theory*. New York: Oxford University Press, Inc.

Zheng, X. (2016a) Dose correction in medical X-ray imaging at low dose regime. *Journal of Medical Imaging and Health Informatics*. 6(7), pp. 1818–1822.

Zheng, X. (2016b) Attenuation based governing equations for automatic exposure and peak voltage controls in medical X-ray CT imaging. *CT Theory and Applications*. 25(6), pp.625–632.

Zheng, X. (2017a) Patient size based guiding equations for automatic mAs and kVp selections in general medical X-ray projection radiography. *Radiation Protection Dosimetry.* 174(4), pp. 545–550.

Zheng, X. (2017b) General equations for optimal selection of diagnostic image acquisition parameters in clinical X-ray imaging. *Radiological Physics and Technology.* 10(4), pp. 415–421.

Zheng, X. (2018) Patient size and tube voltage dependent guiding equations for optimal selection of image acquisition parameters in clinical X-ray imaging. *Radiological Physics and Technology.* 11(2), pp. 212–218.

Zheng, X.M. and Smith, P.V. (1991). The structure of the diamond (111) surface – A SLAB-MINDO study. *Surface Science* 253, pp. 395–404.

Zheng, X.M. and Williams, R.C. (2002) On serum caffeine levels after 24 hours abstention: Clinical implications on Dipyridamole-Thallium-201 myocardial perfusion imaging. *Journal of Nuclear Medicine Technology* 30, pp. 123–127.

Zheng, X.M., Gifford, H.C., Pretorius, P.H. and King, M.A. (2003) An observer study of reconstruction strategies for the detection of solitary pulmonary nodules using hybrid NeoTect SPECT images. *IEEE Nuclear Science Symposium and Medical Imaging Conference Record.* 4, pp. 2690–2694.

Zheng, X.M., Zubal, I.G., Seibyl, J.P. and King, M.A. (2004) Correction for scatter and cross-talk contaminations in dual radionuclide 99m-Tc and 123-I images using artificial neural network. *IEEE Transactions on Nuclear Science* 51(5), pp. 2649–2653.

Zheng, X., Kim, T.M., Davidson, R., Lee, S., Shin, C. and Sook Yang, S. (2014). CT X-ray tube voltage optimization and image reconstruction evaluation using visual grading analysis. *Proceedings of SPIE (Medical Imaging).* 9033, p. 903328.

Zheng, X., Kim, T.M., Sook Yang, S. and Kim, Y. (2015). Studies of CT system performances using visual grading scaling: A methodological comparison among visual grading characteristics, ordinal regression and logistic psychometric functions. *International Journal of Computer Assisted Radiology and Surgery* 10 (Suppl. 1), pp. S5–S6.

Zheng, X., Kim, T.M. and Yang, S. (2016) Optimal kVp in chest computed radiography using visual grading scores: A comparison between visual grading characteristics and ordinal regression analysis. *Proceedings of SPIE (Medical Imaging).* 9783, pp. 97836A1–97836A8.

Zheng, X., Chiang, H-W., Li, J-H., Chiang, H-J., and Lin, L-H. (2018) Personal exposure prescription method reduces dose in radiography. *Radiologic Technology.* 89(5), pp. 435–440.

Zheng, X., Al-Hayek, Y., Cummins, C., Li, X., Nardi, L., Albari, K., Evans, J., Roworth, E. and Seaton, T. (2020) Body size and tube voltage dependent corrections for Hounsfield Unit in medical X-ray computed tomography: Theory and experiments. *Scientific Reports.* 10, p. 15696.

8 Qualitative Approaches for Radiography

Christopher M. Hayre

8.1 INTRODUCTION

This chapter examines common qualitative research designs that have been applied in radiography. By introducing these, it seeks to offer some foundational knowledge and understanding as to why they may be used, with clear signposting to seminal texts. It is generally accepted that more qualitative research is needed in our profession, to not only capture our day-to-day practices and behaviours, but also understand the reasoning, attitudes and actions of practitioners (Bolderston, 2014). There is the suggestion that radiography is struggling, in part, to apply its evidence *in* practice (Snaith, 2016) and later discussed via the utility of action research, in response to change management strategies, and how it may pave the way for translating evidence-based knowledge into the everyday space.

Although radiography has historically been closely aligned to positivism, with medicine, qualitative research is becoming widely recognized and applied, in response to its originality (Bleiker et al., 2019). The positivist and quantitative tradition, however, remains central in light of our continuing need for dose optimization, for instance. As a researcher who appreciates the value of each paradigmatic tradition, the qualitative and quantitative debacle is henceforth viewed mutually and collegially. There is a contrary argument whereby positivistic outlooks may even be indoctrinated and viewed as 'the superior methodology'. Whilst this may lead to a unilateral positivistic ideology within our profession, qualitative research may be challenged or possibly opposed by some, as observed in the other literature (Howard, 2016). Whilst, at present, this is not generally the case, there is recognition that both natural and social science approaches will continue to develop our knowing and understanding in order to enhance 'what radiographers do and how they do it' (Adams and Smith, 2003, p.194).

This chapter can help students or practitioners understand more about qualitative research methodologies if engaging in the topic for the first time, especially if thinking about undertaking a qualitative study. For instance, do you think your study benefits from being ethnographic or grounded theory? Being able to discern the differences can shed light on whether ethnography is the appropriate methodology of choice, or perhaps best suited to grounded theory? Whilst this chapter and other literature

DOI: 10.1201/9780367559311-8

within and outside of radiography tends to focus on forthcoming methodologies as merely qualitative, there is a growing trend for approaches to incorporate quantitative methods, both outside and within radiography. It is strongly recommended that readers continue to challenge and think about alternate methodological models via this complimentary lens of incorporating quantitative methods, if deemed appropriate. For now, however, and for the purposes of this book and its undergraduate audience, convention will remain the primary focus.

8.2   THE VALUE OF QUALITATIVE APPROACHES

The ultimate aim of all research is to seek or find new information. When teaching research methods to students I begin by accepting that our search for 'truth' is perhaps elusive and abstract in all research. Even in the most controlled X-ray experiment. By recognizing this, it attempts to reaffirm the view that either qualitative or quantitative methods may suit the needs of the research question(s) and also offer an informed view about what it is they wish to find out. For instance, some students may try to pursue quantitative research in light of seeking 'truth', to do something 'groundbreaking' or 'breath-taking' (as I intended at the beginning of my PhD study). Yet, in reality, the research idea/question could be best explored by qualitative research and offer greater insight to the profession. The importance and value of qualitative research in radiography, then, is to provide unique and deep-rooted insights to help uncover undocumented findings amongst individuals or a group (Denzin, 1997). Looking back from a philosophical standpoint in chapter 2, we appreciate that qualitative research is not trying to generalize our reality but to uncover 'multiple realities' of those members within a particular group (Benton and Craib, 2001). This provides us with an alternate dimension to what 'truth' may mean for some, based on our/their ontology and thus conform to what is commonly regarded as a specific 'research tradition'. For example, the first author [CH] has engaged in qualitative and quantitative methodologies, the former utilizing ethnography (Hayre et al., 2019) and grounded theory (Benfield, Hewis and Hayre, 2021) and latter examining dose optimization via X-ray experimentation (Hayre et al., 2018a; Hayre, Jeffery and Bungay, 2020). This interchangeable use has been developed because of the self-development and self-actualization of ethnography alone and how qualitative and quantitative methods play a pivotal role in this methodology, attributing it to the role of radiographers (Hayre et al., in press). As mentioned above, it will also have implications for disciplines in order to help evolve and develop research methodologies based on research questions.

Qualitative research shares a common theme whereby it seeks to share the lived experience of individuals as they, themselves not only play a critical role in the world around them but offer insight into the lived experiences concerning specific events. Across most qualitative work, the theory of shared symbolic interactionism by Goffman (1968) remains a key feature. Goffman recognized human adaptation and communication as being pivotal within our environment(s) (ibid). Further, the concept of symbolism can be shared across objects, events, or protocols within which a particular group shares. For instance, in radiography, the X-ray tube is a commonly shared 'tool' and thus by symbolizing its prevalence in the clinical context, we can understand its application, facilitation and limitation. Further, this adaptation within the qualitative setting is continuously evolving because whilst previous qualitative papers may highlight insights surrounding dose optimization or patient care, it does not mean its empirical value remains contemporary. It could be argued that the success of its empirical value is via critical engagement with its readers, which in turn helps limit the issue altogether. Whilst possible, it does demonstrate that qualitative data and the context in which it is captured will evolve over time due to alternate social and technological practices. A central component, argued here, is that qualitative research should evolve because like our everyday world, social change surrounds us whereby our adaptation and responses to emerging change remain necessary.

A key component of qualitative research is its ability to explore events in the 'natural setting'. At first glance, we should not confuse this with the 'natural sciences' via naturalistic forms of enquiry, i.e., atoms, molecules and/or X-ray photons. Qualitative research uses the term 'naturalistic' to reinforce the natural order in a society or culture, i.e., the everyday social-cultural practice of a mammography department. This form of naturalistic enquiry may be culturally specific or have a specific phenomenon. Yet, for the qualitative researcher, there is always the challenge of capturing natural events, with themselves remaining the instrument. This is discussed in more detail below and later in chapter 9.

It is important to highlight that it is not within the scope of this chapter to try and problem-solve the abovementioned debates – there are already a number of useful publications that seek to address this (see Guba and Lincoln, 1994; Griffiths and Norman, 2013). However, a quick observation of metrics of readers transnationally for my own qualitative and quantitative paper highlights an interesting outcome. Upon comparison of qualitative (non-generalizable) outputs with quantitative (generalizable) papers, there is greater interest (at the time of writing this book, at least) with qualitative outputs (Hayre, 2016a; Hayre, 2016b), when compared, say, to quantitative and 'more generalizable' work (Hayre et al., 2018a; Mercado and Hayre, 2018). In addition, a qualitative paper was used in the development of policy upon considering the application and use of lead protection in general radiography (Hayre et al., 2017). Here, there is some insight that quantitative approaches may not favorably inform policy decisions in diagnostic radiography or demonstrate 'greater impact' for the profession. Moreover, it supports previous assertions that greater need and justification for qualitative research can enable us to understand the practice and professional behaviour of radiographic practice and perhaps have a greater impact in years to come.

A primary feature of all qualitative research stems from the level of depth required to understand a topic or concept well. The advantages of qualitative research can be profound, not just from an empirical perspective but also as a self-development tool. Although we may not typically attribute qualitative research with generalization (as expected in the scientific sense), some generalization is still plausible, depending on the group, policy decision-making or managers to whom the findings resonate. In my view, if data resonates with practitioners and academics internationally, then its purpose is not to seek 'empirical generalizability' but 'wider cultural identifiability' as it is not the data *per se* that seeks to be generalized, but a wider appreciation and value for its audience. This can be readily transferred not only via dissemination but also via clinical and academic teachings/conversations and/or between everyday communications with individuals, pervading conventional metrics. We should also acknowledge that qualitative studies provide description(s) of undocumented findings within a specific context of the inquiry and thus has importance amongst the researcher(s). Notably, this may become the rationale for selecting a qualitative methodology by uncovering what has previously been seen or heard within the workplace. This leads us to acknowledge that our close encounters with topics, contexts and colleagues remain unique, in which qualitative research seeks to evidence. Importantly, if we decided to use different researchers, but perform the same study on the same participants, in the same location, and at the same time, it is likely the final analysis and write-up will differ. Whilst it may be assumed that identical themes will arise, this is unlikely. Although some themes or aspects will be similar as researchers attribute more value to specific outcomes due to their own axiology, it may also lead to alternate forms of knowledge in respect to the epistemological framework. This does not mean that qualitative research is invalid or untrustworthy – later examined in Chapter 10. It simply recognizes individuality and diversity, which are captured and examined upon ensuring the trustworthiness of qualitative research. This enables subsequent readers to critique interpretations made by the researcher, which can be traced back, supported with existential tools to help reinforce empirical findings.

The utilization of inductive reasoning, as a 'bottom up' approach in qualitative research seeks to uncover new radiography phenomena that has little empirical insight. The utility of inductive reasoning allows a researcher to discover evidence that is embryonic, unique and/or even challenge/break down current ideological norms. This is perhaps a key rationale for pursuing this type of research because whereas radiography has stemmed from positivism, there remains a lack of insight, openness or critique into how radiographers behave and apply knowledge. This 'closed' and underexplored nature remains its limitation, yet with qualitative work becoming increasingly used, coupled with innovative methodologies, we are beginning to challenge the status quo and question our cultural and practical norms by ensuring practice behaviours remain grounded on sound evidence.

A key feature of all qualitative research resides in its interpretative component about the world around us, whereby data is often based on verbatim, rather than numerical representation. The former is a powerful tool either via observation or simply listening to members of that community. Further, the versatility of methodological strategies does not need to be prescribed, unlike X-ray experiments, which requires controlled and rigorous conditions in order enhance both reliability and validity. In some parts, whilst this chapter provides insight, it also celebrates the attributes of qualitative research for prospective researchers in the field of radiography, which will now be discussed. The four methodologies, as mentioned at the beginning will now be discussed.

8.3   ETHNOGRAPHY

Ethnography is 'positioned' here under the qualitative heading because there is the general acceptance it aligns with this research paradigm. Bronislaw Malinowski is considered the father of ethnography, establishing the importance of first-hand participant observation of everyday life, which is now essential in this methodological strategy. Malinowski, through his travels, notably Australia, led him to the practice of participant observation and his seminal book, *Argonauts of the Western Pacific* (Malinowski, 1984). Following its publication, Malinowski became a well-regarded anthropologist in the world of ethnography. When we think about ethnography, then, it closely resembles participant observation and still remains its distinguishing feature when compared to other research designs (ibid).

Before we examine ethnographic research in radiography, we should first consider its uses in other disciplines in order to help contextualize the need for its approach. For instance, ethnography has been used in politics, sociology and business and now found its uses in education and healthcare (Hammersley and Atkinson, 2007). In education, ethnography has been used to understand student life in elementary and high schools. Examples of ethnographic research range from examining the student–teacher relationship (Praag, Stevens and Houtte, 2017) and also via community-based subjects (Nichols et al., 2017). Ethnography has become generally accepted in the fields of nursing and medicine, leading to an array of novel empiricism, including cancer diagnosis (The et al., 2000), and doctor/nurse–patient relationships in acute hospital setting (Strauss et al., 1963). In short, the role of ethnography is grounded on the belief that it is the behaviour and culture of groups or sub-groups that influence a setting in which education and/or healthcare takes place.

In radiography, then, the use of ethnography has evolved in the last 10–15 years. There is now a firm body of evidence, which has captured unique insights by different researchers (Larsson et al., 2007; Strudwick, 2015; Nightingale et al., 2016; Hayre, 2016a). Ethnography can be readily distinguished amongst other qualitative methodologies due to its investigation into a culture or sub-culture. As Malinowski sought to examine the cultural life of Aboriginal Australians, via participant immersion and observation, ethnography is able to provide deep cultural accounts of its members, including radiographers. For radiography, understanding the culture of its members is critical to determine what it is they are thinking or doing in their professional capacity. This can only be achieved through immersion via observing radiographers within their natural setting, i.e., the X-ray room or communal viewing area, as depicted in Figure 8.1. Whilst participant observation remains key, other qualitative methods are used to support and/or refute observations made by researchers, discussed further in chapter 9. These may include interviewing, examination of documents, reflective journals, surveys (and/or X-ray experiments). These are tools (methods) that can be used to help triangulate evidence in order to build a better picture of, say, computed tomography (CT) practice.

The 'attendance' of the researcher remains an important feature when it comes to collecting data. Because participant observation enables researchers to see 'what is happening' and 'how it's happening', this may not always take place in the X-ray room. Although the X-ray room may be the primary area of data generation, ethnography also takes the researcher to other environments, i.e., the staff room or viewing area. Less formal environments can elicit different responses from participants, whether over lunch or tea/coffee breaks. It also attributes less clinical urgency and possibly less intrusion by the researcher. In short, the role of the ethnographer and

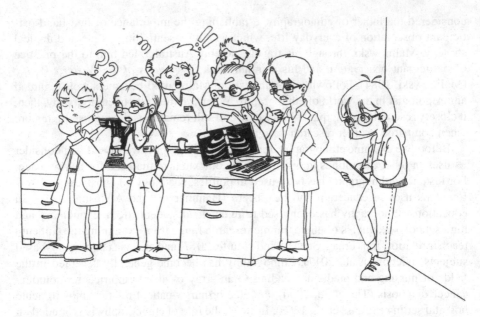

FIGURE 8.1   The observation of radiographers in practice.

use of participant observation provides experiences grounded upon the participant's everyday actions, behaviours and attitudes of the phenomena under examination (Hammersley and Atkinson, 2007), in which the culture takes place.

In radiology, there are still few contemporary studies that ethnographically explore CT), magnetic resonance imaging (MRI) or ultrasonography, for instance. There is a greater need and opportunity for prospective researchers to perform ethnographies in these settings in order to document areas of consideration. The abovementioned modalities remain technologically focused but require human input from radiographers to perform and optimize scanning parameters to meet clinical and patient needs. Further, even if technological and physical principles are understood, it may be its application, integration or operation of such principles that are misunderstood. This is central in ethnographic work when compared to other qualitative methodologies.

Ethnography requires prolonged engagement by researchers, although there is growing acceptance of 'rapid ethnographies' (Vindrola-Padros, 2021). It is pertinent that researchers observe and interact over a period of time that requires close affiliation, knowledge and understanding regarding the topic of interest. Thus to become 'an ethnographer' or 'ethno-radiographer' as previously termed, researchers should spend sufficient time with their participants in their natural setting to understand and learn from the culture of interest. This is important because ethnography is based on the assumption that what people say and practice is being consciously or unconsciously moulded by the behaviours of others. In turn, this requires sensitivity amongst the researcher whereby he/she's initial questions, persona, attire and prior relationships are crafted in order for the understudy to welcome and, importantly, accept the researcher. These ongoing interactions with participants enhance rapport, which attempts to yield better responses or 'more natural' observations/responses. A common concept in most overt observations is the Hawthorne effect, whereby radiographers will deliberately react positively upon being observed (Burgess, 1993). However, in time, it is generally accepted that such reactive behaviour fades leading to the 'true' behaviour emerging over a period of prolonged engagement (ibid). In short, whilst a limitation of ethnographic work, whereby actors alter behaviours in the clinical context, however, recognition that the Hawthorne effect can be mitigated against and continuously reflected upon by the researcher is captured by patterns of behaviour that may be seen as inferior by others.

Data collection methods are far-reaching and typically involve participant observation, interviewing, analysis of documents and/or the analysis of images or photos. However, a critical and often undisclosed element of data collection resides with participant observation. For instance, from experience of conducting ethnographic observations, it is not uncommon to collect verbal narratives between participants (or indirectly with patients); a collection of verbal communications between the researcher and participants; nonverbal behaviour, i.e., the action of moving X-ray equipment or transferring a patient onto the X-ray table; aspects of the environment which require an action of those which did not receive action or attention – a patient calling for assistance or the decision to disclose a patients diagnosis, upon request. As this suggests, there are a number of 'empirical events' that take place during observational fieldwork, which cannot be captured via one-to-one interviewing. What will remain essential is that researchers reflect on their questions and deem what is necessary to collect for the purposes of initial research questions, as outlined by the literature review and gap analysis.

Ethnography has played a critical role for many disciplines and is now demonstrating significance both methodologically and empirically in radiography. In short, as researchers in radiography, we are finely poised between the natural and social sciences. Whilst ethnography typically applies qualitative methods to observe and enquire into radiographic behaviour, there is the opportunity, in radiography, to incorporate experimental research. This is grounded on participant observation that paves the way for encompassing two distinct research paradigms within a single methodological strategy and captures the day-to-day practices and experiences of radiographers and patients alike.

8.4   PHENOMENOLOGY

Phenomenology is another philosophical perspective applicable to the social sciences. It is generally linked to Edmund Husserl, who, at the time, turned away from the traditional positivistic appeals derived from scientific constructs and sought to capture the human experience of the 'things themselves', which we consider 'phenomena' (Husserl, 2010). The identification and acknowledgement of these beliefs must be recognized, which is often referred as the 'epoche process' (ibid). Husserl believed that intentionality, the significance of being present in a given situation, contained both a noema (perception) and a noesis (meaning). There are three main tenets to phenomenology that have emerged over the years; transcendental, existential and hermeneutic (Laverty, 2003). An example of transcendental research in radiography could be 'what are the experiences of patients undergoing MRI imaging with claus-trophobia'? An existential phenomenology, however, would ask a different question, such as 'how do radiographers perceive patients with claustrophobia whilst under-going MRI procedures'? Lastly, hermeneutic phenomenology examines language and communication, thus offer the following question: what have radiographers and patients learned about claustrophobia during MRI imaging? The phenomenological approach involves confronting a particular experience (like claustrophobia in MRI) but provides comprehensive description(s) that accurately illustrates the nature of the experience (from whichever perspective is necessary). It is important, then, that any preconceived ideas, about claustrophobia from the researcher, are 'stripped back' when examining results. Having experienced MRI as a radiographer (and a patient), this would be important to acknowledge. Throughout the research, prior thoughts and assumptions or experiences should be recognized in order to prevent the researcher's own biases from overshadowing essential descriptions. Colaizzi (1973) affirms this asserting that the phenomenologist's role is to accurately describe phenomena that is seen through the eyes of his or her participants by asking pertinent questions concerning the research topic itself.

Scholars working with phenomenological traditions assert that social scientists cannot fully understand human behaviour without understanding the framework within which the subjects interpret their thoughts, feelings and actions (Colaizzi, 1973). Hence, the requirement for researchers to achieve a 'transcendental state', which seeks to move beyond our own preconceived ideas (epoche) to see phenomena through unclouded glasses, leading to greater meaning of the phenomena (Laverty, 2003). The intention by Husserl was evident, to establish a theory of knowledge, free of presuppositions and assumptions of any worldview, including those traditional principles of logic confined by the natural sciences (Husserl, 2010). This philosoph-ical perspective propelled the phenomenological methodology because it proffered an approach that was able to overcome barriers associated with observational methods, as seen with ethnography for instance. It could be argued, then, that phenomenological research allows researchers to specifically derive radiographic empiricism about phe-nomena through direct interaction with participants and via non-assumptive means.

Phenomenology has been used in radiography and continues to offer important and novel insights for researchers. Murphy et al. (2015) investigated compression behaviours of practitioners during mammographic screening. The researchers used six focus group interviews with practitioners, coincided with six one-to-one interviews with educators. Lundvall et al. (2014) sought to examine radiographer's experi-ence of professional work using a combination of interviews and observations using interpretative phenomenology. The authors identified that radiographers considered patient safety, coupled with their own knowledge and skill to provide optimal images, which remained central in the clinical space. These examples demonstrate the util-ization of phenomenology in order to focus on specific practice-based phenomena. In my view, phenomenology offers inductive approaches to underexplored radiographic phenomena and linked with a specific focus, unified by how the world appears to those individuals experiencing it.

Phenomenological research is interested in the subjective experiences of participants seeking to unravel how participants come to experience similar understandings of the world, often termed inter-subjectivity (Laverty, 2003). Amongst phenomenologists, it was felt possible to observe reality in its genuine form via phenomenological research, especially if preconceived ideas are removed and/or distanced (Koopman, 2015). Moving forward, for any prospective researcher seeking to utilize phenomenology, researchers need to clarify information pertinent to the phenomenon itself, such as an area within an imaging modality, a patient's experience, or something experienced as a student. The researchers' overall aim should be to provide a deep, contextual lens of the phenomena as 'real-life' from the lived experiences of those individuals whom are experiencing it. The 'lived experience' is something that phenomenologists seek to determine through critical evaluation of appropriate research methods (Laverty, 2003). As previously discussed, for ethnography, phenomenology can take many forms, and whilst examples in the literature focus on qualitative approaches, studies elsewhere have demonstrated the integration of quantitative methods, supporting phenomena pertinent to a specific discipline (Fisher and Stenner, 2014).

As a researcher applying phenomenology, it offers a number of advantages. This can range from examining memories, thoughts, instincts, emotions and desires. Further, in terms of engagement with radiography, phenomenology seeks to examine consciousness and thus accounts for a plethora of experiences that can be accounted for, including self-experience, awareness of others, linguistic activity and the everyday actions in our radiography environment. Key to the practice of phenomenology is that of hermeneutics, the art of interpretation in context, in particular, social and linguistic cues.

8.5 GROUNDED THEORY

Glaser and Strauss are recognized as the founders of grounded theory research. Glaser was conversant with descriptive statistics, with Strauss, symbolic interactionism. The collaborative efforts amongst these researchers enabled critical examination of terminally ill patients who identified alternate knowledge and opinions concerning their health status (Glaser and Strauss, 1965). For instance, some patients whom suspected they were dying tried to prove or disprove their suspicions, whereas, for others, some tried to infer their prognosis by interpreting the treatment of caregivers and/or family members (ibid). This seminal work examined how patients dealt with the knowledge of death and also reactions felt by healthcare workers. During their work, authors questioned the appropriateness and use of the scientific method as a means of verification, leading to the constant comparative method, a key feature in grounded theory research. This is outlined in their text *Awareness of Dying (1965)* (ibid). Their later publication laid the foundations for the grounded theory methodology, titled *The Discovery of Grounded Theory* (Glaser and Strauss, 1999). In this text, we appreciate that whilst grounded theory is structured (as with all methodologies for replication), it also remains flexible if very little is known about a concept (ibid). This approach has been found useful in work undertaken in Australia (Benfield, Hewis and Hayre, 2021), the examination of the phenomena 'dose creep' amongst a cohort of undergraduate radiography students. The lack of literature surrounding this topic is generally recognized amongst student cohorts but has implications for students and radiographers. For instance, it highlights challenges not only from a workforce standpoint but also from an educational aspect, both academically and clinically. In response to the few studies concerning this topic, the rationale for utilising grounded theory was deemed appropriate by enabling the examination of this topic amongst an underrepresented group. The study sought to lay the foundations for the delivery of student radiographer learning, and although six participants took part, the knowledge and insight gained provides an embryonic platform for future work. Whilst other grounded theory models have been used, earlier studies also offer critical insight into this methodology. Walsh (2010), for instance, discusses the role of grounded theory within the radiotherapy profession and in particular with cancer patients. The author highlights that grounded theory offered unique and descriptive accounts of cancer pathway experiences amongst patients and provided vital empiricism for future work. Other studies applying grounded theory methodologies focused on coping strategies developed by children who had not previously undergone MRI examinations (Kada et al., 2018). Kada et al (2018) used 22 semi-structured interviews with children immediately after undergoing an MRI procedure. Sevens and Reeves (2019) later looked at barriers to employing sonographer graduates using grounded theory, highlighting future developments and requirements. As evidenced, the use of grounded theory seeks to play a key role in providing impactful critiques to underrepresented concepts and offers a way of deconstructing or challenging perceptions, whilst facilitating discovery-orientated empiricism.

The utility of grounded theory is again based on sparse empirical evidence for a given context or concept and as noted with other qualitative approaches, grounded theory utilizes symbolic interactionism (Tie, Birks and Francis, 2019). In our grounded theory work, we uncovered how 'dose creep' remained heavily influenced by academic lecturers, clinical supervisors, misinformation and perception (Benfield, Hewis and Hayre, 2021). Thus, the objects, peers and 'evidence' in which students are typically exposed remained accountable to the practice of dose creep for graduating radiographers. In short, grounded theory is not simply a methodology used by researchers but also an outcome of a project whereby 'theory' is 'grounded' by the research participants themselves.

In later years following the discovery of the grounded theory, Glaser and Strauss began to disagree around some aspects of grounded theory and later wrote independently. Glaser in 1987 published his book on *Theoretical Sensitivity (1978)* (Glaser, 1978) and Strauss later publishing *Qualitative Analysis for Social Scientists (1987)* (Strauss, 1987). The paper by Rennie (1998) offers a sound critique for assessing the divergence of these two prominent scholars and useful for prospective researchers seeking historical development of grounded theory. The often stark contradiction between the two prominent academics remained philosophical (ibid). Today, however, we now observe different alterations and philosophical perspectives to grounded theory, which can also include interpretivism and postmodernism, offering different ways of uncovering new knowledge.

Charmaz (2006) helps define grounded theory a little further identifying it as a method of conducting qualitative research that focuses on creating conceptual frameworks or theories through building inductive analysis from the data. Glaser (1978) acknowledged that the goal of classic grounded theory is by generating a conceptual theory that accounts for a pattern of behaviour relevant and problematic to those involved. These perspectives are important in radiography research because there is still little known about our own practices, 'ways of doing things' and phenomena regularly discussed. Further, because the evidence is still emerging, coupled with an inherent interconnectivity with technology, natural sciences and social sciences, this will arguably create an array of theoretical occurrences now and in future years.

Because grounded theory is typically aligned to the qualitative research paradigm and often regarded as structured, albeit flexible, the selection of grounded theory is often appropriate when little is known about a particular concept. Grounded theory, then, constructs theory 'grounded' on the everyday area of enquiry in order to provide valued insight. At the time, Glaser and Strauss (1965) were challenging the empirical validity of qualitative approaches, but now it remains widely utilized in a number of health-based disciplines, and will continue to play a crucial role in the development of evidence-based knowledge.

8.6   ACTION RESEARCH

Action research is considered a qualitative research design; however, it separates itself from the abovementioned approaches by recognizing its ability to 'liberate' and be 'life-enhancing' (MacDonald, 2012, p.35). There are a number of other terms that action research is also recognized by; 'participatory action research', 'participatory research' and 'community-based participatory research' (Holkup et al., 2004). Hereafter, it is referred as 'action research'. The origins of action research are generally attributed to Kurt Lewin (1946), a Prussian psychologist and Jewish refugee of Nazi Germany. His philosophy affirmed that people would be more motivated if they were involved in both decision-making and workplace reform (Hussain et al., 2018). A keyword here is 'workplace', and thus, the work of Lewin is often associated with organizational/workplace change, vis-à-vis, change management processes (ibid). However, it also has value in healthcare and to researchers seeking to impose some form of change in the workplace. For example, a researcher may desire to change a form of fluoroscopic practice, for the betterment of patient care, dose optimization or reporting of images, leading to an improved outcome(s).

Action research is a methodology that facilitates the business model by remaining client/customer focused in order to solve social problems. There are several stages recognized within the action research framework by Lewin, which include observation, reflection, action [implementation], evaluation and modification (Lewin, 1946). The rationale for incorporating action research is in response to involving participants that are perhaps 'oppressed' or unable to voice their concerns about an underrepresented issue (Baum, MacDougall and Smith, 2006). This type of research methodology, then, as captured in chapter 2 could be aligned with postmodernism whereby those who remain underrepresented are given a voice in order for change to be actioned. This also includes the development of a critical consciousness of research participants, whereby improvement to the lives of those participating in the process remains paramount, coincided with the transformation of societal structures or relationships, helping facilitate change. For radiography, this may manifest in our ability to 'get close' to participants, within which a topic resides. Upon data collection, if the researcher identifies an area of change, for example, the protection of privacy and dignity amongst patients undergoing a fluoroscopic procedure, then he/she may implement a strategy using existing workplace structures and work with senior staff to implement change. As part of this process, the researcher may lean towards being a participant, a facilitator or learner in the process. Reflection is important in the change process whereby review and re-evaluation are needed (ibid). This is critical because change may not be successful in light of social-cultural aspects; naturally, such change may resonate with one environment but not applicable to others (Fiedler, 1964). The consideration of change brought about by the research process should be viewed critically in light of the values held by patients or radiographers. It is recognized these will differ depending on the culture (local or national), in which action research captures the constraints of their own political, economic and social contexts.

The principle purpose of action research is the creation of social change; it also seeks to unlock the capacity for decision-making of individuals, i.e., the patients voice, who perhaps remain underrepresented in radiography. The obvious juxtaposition here is that patients remain at the centre and the driving force behind any betterment of radiographic work. Typically, then, in order 'break out' and challenge the language, action or interactions with patients undergoing fluoroscopic examinations, the researcher may yield postmodernism, whereby conventional norms surrounding privacy and dignity are challenged with alternate ways of thinking or doing are applied. This also suggests the 'action researcher' remains on a self-educative journey via social investigation, which leads to practice improvement by taking action within the clinical environment. This type of methodological inquiry and action-focused approach segregates itself with other qualitative designs as it intends to impose some practical change management in the context under examination.

There have been a number of action research methodologies carried out in radiography. For instance, Barlow and Owens (2018) sought to investigate an open access (walk-in) service in radiography, in order to reduce waiting times. The authors reflected upon surrounding hospitals to whom had implemented this type of radiological service. The study sought the opinions of radiology managers and radiography staff using semi-structured interviews and focus groups. In the same year, Naylor and Foulkes (2018) investigated radiographers working in the operating theatre with onus on developing, piloting and sustaining simulation for radiography students to assist with interprofessional skills. Their action-based simulation project provided a valuable tool for prospective radiographers, to whom would struggle with theatre radiography upon graduation. Here, this identifies how action-based research remains central for educationalists in radiography by improving educational experiences, as well as preparing students for the workplace.

Action research is specifically linked to a discipline with intentions of *informing* and *changing* practices for the future. Whilst recognised in education as a way of engaging, reflecting and improving a student's behaviour/experience, radiography is now witnessing its use to help inform and change the way practice is delivered. The concept of action research begins with researchers posing a set of research questions, gather the necessary data, reflect and then decide on a course of action. The final component, the desire to change an existing course of action, is what sets aside action research from other qualitative research designs. As previously highlighted, whilst the abovementioned methodologies seek to add to the existing evidence by examining a culture or sub-culture, specific phenomena, or data 'grounded' on individuals, they arguably seek to impart change outside the methodological context, either via dissemination or via policy development. Further, whilst additional questions, ideas and other forms of enquiry may be uncovered as part of this process, it is focused on seeking original knowledge to improve a situation, skills and/or strategies. On the other hand, action research may not overtly be interested in learning why or how we do certain things in a particular way, but rather on how 'things' can be altered for the betterment of radiographic services.

A limitation of action research, when compared to other qualitative studies is often attributed to its longitudinal approach whereby the researcher is required to spend prolonged time within the environment (Bergold and Thomas, 2012). For example, if the study is being conducted over a prolonged period of time, participants that were involved in a study may have moved to different organizations and/or perhaps transitioned into other imaging specialties (ibid). Whilst this may also occur in other qualitative designs, the often prolonged engagement in the research field should remain a consideration for prospective methodological designs amongst prospective researchers. Other methodological aspects for consideration resonate with overcoming and deconstructing 'what is currently performed', requiring egalitarian motives. It is generally recognised that any form of change management can bring about uncertainty amongst its members. Thus, if a superintendent radiographer or radiology manager decides to perform action research amongst his/her colleagues, then considerations surrounding cohesion and confirmation bias must be considered prior to engaging participants. There is an obvious imbalance of power whereby a senior staff member seeks to question junior staff in participating in a prospective study in order to impact some form of change, as previously highlighted in chapter 4.

There is also a clear advantage in relation to action research for prospective researchers in our contemporary space. In light of the possibility that existing evidence fails to be properly implemented clinically, this type of methodology may help interconnect theory with practice as a change management tool to help build and impart evidence in our clinical work. We must also remind ourselves that the purpose of radiographic research is for the betterment of patient treatment, management and care, rather than simply the production of knowledge. Thus failing to impart new knowledge in order to facilitate patient outcomes will arguably require further action. In education, for instance, action research has been found useful by informing pedagogical outcomes (UDAS, 1998), thus if such strategies are used, either from a research or managerial perspective, it may enable radiographers to act on evidence. The principle of action-based radiography, whilst may be occurring whereby radiographers use reflection or reflexivity as a tool for thinking about improvement, there is perhaps now a greater need for a more formal strategy to actually impart some workplace change.

If action research remains limited there are some practical components, even if anecdotal. For instance, it may resonate with superintendent radiographers or radiology managers as there will always be change management decisions taking place. Further, although research may not be the focus, the principle and practice of action research may still be useful as an implementation strategy. For formal action research, then, it does offer researchers and practitioners a line of inquiry that carefully plans, executes and critically reflects on changes made in order to generate solutions to existing radiographic problems, coupled with its ability to empower members of the radiographic community, and above all else, benefit patients.

8.7 CHAPTER SUMMARY

This chapter has provided insight into four generally recognized methodological strategies primarily aligned to qualitative research. The chapter began by setting the scene discussing the value of qualitative approaches in radiography and how they have and will continue to challenge and add value to our profession. Ethnography, phenomenology, grounded theory and action research were discussed, linking to contemporary radiographic literature. The primary purpose of this chapter has been to not only highlight these methodologies, with appropriate signposting to seminal works but to understand the core values of each. This chapter has deliberately not elaborated on the research 'methods' or 'tools' within this chapter. These are outlined descriptively next in chapter 9 because choices of methods may not only differ but may be used interchangeably depending on the methodology. At this stage, there has been no deliberate attempt to prescribe methodological approaches in order for readers to keep questioning. What is important, at present, is the recognition, value and application of qualitative research designs and how they continue to contribute to radiographic practice. By encapsulating these frameworks, it is expected that students can learn and understand some advantages and disadvantages of each, which is ultimately driven by emerging research questions and the discovery of originality.

KEY TERMS

Action research: a research methodology generally applied in the social sciences by applying transformative change throughout the methodological process.

Anthropologist: is a person engaged in the practice of anthropology, which is the study of humans, the norms and values in society.

Culture: Is commonly regarded as the ideas, customs and social behaviour of a particular people or society.

Discourse: is a written or spoken communication of debate.

Epoché process: is commonly referred to as 'bracketing' in phenomenological research and used as a process to block biases or assumptions in order to describe a phenomenon in terms of its own inherent system of meaning.

Ethnography: is the study of the scientific description of a people and their culture with their customs, habits and mutual differences noted.

Evidence: is an available body of information indicating whether a belief or proposition is valid.

Grounded theory: is regarded as a systematic methodology that has typically been applied to qualitative research. It is also a methodology that has flexibility in its application in a number of social science settings.

Hawthorne effect: is a phenomenon whereby participants in a study react to and then modify an aspect of their behaviour in response to being observed.

Ideology: a system of ideas and beliefs and is usually linked to political theory. It also has relevance in sociology and can be applied to other disciplines, such as radiography.

Inductive reasoning: is a method of reasoning to supply evidence, generally through observation and generally assumes probabilistic outcomes.

Interpretivism: is involved in researchers interpreting elements of the study, thus interpretivism integrates human interest into a study and also acknowledges differences between social actors in a single study.

Longitudinal: is typically referred to as a research design over a long period of time. It can be used in a number of qualitative and quantitative methodologies.

Metrics: are quantitative assessments used for tracking of the performance of published research. They are useful for assessing impact, widened participation and visibility transnationally.

Natural setting: is a place where qualitative research takes place. Qualitative researchers, then, study things as they are happening. By researching in the natural setting, qualitative researchers go to the people by gathering sensory data.

Noema: is a word that stems from the Greek word for 'thought', and it is used in phenomenology for the perception and central to the epoché process.

Noesis: is closely linked to classical philosophy, which is closely resembled to intellect or intelligence.

Phenomenology: is the philosophical study of the structures of experience itself. It concentrates on the study of consciousness and the objects of direct experience.

Policymaking: is a policy stemming from a deliberate system of principles to guide decisions and achieve rational outcomes. A policy is a statement of intent and is implemented as a procedure or protocol.

Sub-culture: a cultural group within a large cultural group, who often have beliefs or interests at variance with those of the larger group. For instance, a sub-group of MRI radiographers may have differing beliefs concerning patient safety than CT radiographers.

Symbolic interactionism: is a sociological theory developed from practical considerations and developed by words, gestures and other 'symbols' pertinent to the area of exploration.

Trustworthiness: is the ability to be relied upon as honest or truthful.

Verbatim: is used to denote the exact same words as were used originally.

EXERCISES AND STUDY QUESTIONS

1   Before considering a qualitative methodology be mindful of what your intentions are in terms of data generation. Remember, any methodology is like a car engine, it helps you move, progress and importantly allow you to manoeuvre your way through the research field. By reflecting on the four strategies identified here, carefully think and provide a rationale for its use (if applicable), when compared to the other strategies.

2   Whilst research methods will be discussed at some length in the next chapter, try to think about the types of methods you intend to use in your selected methodology. Are these practical, appropriate, and been used elsewhere? Examining previous work is central in understanding the context of your research goals.

3   Qualitative research and methodologies can be useful for finding originality in your line of inquiry. However, do not fully dismiss the use of quantitative methods to help with your project. For those students undertaking higher degree research, there is an opportunity to apply and test innovative and unconventional strategies that seek out new knowledge.

REFERENCES

Adams, J. and Smith, T. (2003) Qualitative methods in radiography research: A proposed framework, *Radiography*, 9(1), pp.193–199.

Baum, F., MacDougall, C., and Smith, D. (2006) Participatory action research. *Journal of Epidemiology and Community Health.* 60(1), pp. 854–857.

Barlow, N., and Owens, M. (2018) Participatory action research into implementing open access in musculoskeletal X-ray: Management and staff perspectives. *Radiography.* 24(3), pp.224–233.

Bergold, J. and Thomas, S. (2012) Participatory research methods: A methodological approach in motion. *Forum Qualitative Sozialforschung.* 13 (1), [Online] Available at: www.qualitative-research.net/index.php/fqs/article/view/1801/3334 (Accessed: 15/03/2021).

Bleiker, J., Morgan-Trimmer, S., Knapp, K., and Hopkins, S. (2019) Navigating the maze: Qualitative research methodologies and their philosophical foundations. *Radiography.* 25(1), pp.S4–S8.

Benfield, S. Hewis, J., and Hayre, C.M. (2021) Investigating perceptions of 'dose creep' amongst student radiographers: A grounded theory study. *Radiography.*

Benton, T. and Craib, I. (2001) *Philosophy of Social Science*, Macmillan: Hampshire

Bolderston, A. (2014) Five percent is not enough! Why we need more qualitative research in the medical radiation sciences. *Journal of Medical Imaging and Radiation Sciences.* 45(1), pp. 201–203.

Burgess, R.G. (1993) *In the Field: Introduction to Field Research*, New York: Routledge.

Charmaz, K. (2006) *Constructing Grounded Theory – A Practice Guide Through Qualitative Analysis.* Thousand Oaks, CA: Sage.

Colaizzi, P.F. (1973) *Reflection and Research in psychology: A Phenomenological Study of Learning.* Dubuque, IA: Kendall/Hunt.

Denzin, N (1997) *Interpretive Ethnography*, London: Sage.

Fiedler, F.E. (1964) A theory of leadership effectiveness. In L. Berkowitz (Ed.), Advances in Experimental Social Psychology. New York: Academic Press.

Fisher, W.P. and Stenner, A.J. (2014) Integrating qualitative and quantitative research approaches via the phenomenological method. *International Journal of Multiple Research Approaches.* 5(1), pp.89–103.

Glaser, B.G. (1978) *Theoretical Sensitivity.* Mill Valley, CA: Sociology Press.

Glaser, B. and Strauss, A. (1965) *Awareness of Dying.* Chicago, IL: Aldine Pub.

Glaser, B.G. and Strauss, A.L. (1999) *Discovery of Grounded Theory – Strategies for Qualitative Researcher.* New Brunswick: Routledge.

Goffman, E. (1968) *Stigma: Notes on the Management of Spoiled Identity.* London: Pelican.

Griffiths, P. and Norman, I. (2013) Qualitative or quantitative? Developing and evaluating complex interventions: Time to end the paradigm war, *International Journal of Nursing Studies,* 50(5), pp.583–584.

Guba, E. G. and Lincoln, Y. S. (1994) Competing paradigms in qualitative research. In Denzin, N.K. and Lincoln, Y.S. (Eds.), *Handbook of Qualitative Research* (pp. 105–117), Thousand Oaks, CA: Sage.

Hammersley, M. and Atkinson, P. (2007) *Ethnography Principles in Practice,* 3rd Edn. New York: Routledge.

Hayre, C.M. Blackman, S. Carlton, K. and Eyden, A. (2017) Attitudes and perceptions of radiographers applying lead (Pb) protection in general radiography. *Radiography.* 24(1), pp. e13–e18.

Hayre, C.M. (2016a) 'Cranking up', 'whacking up' and 'bumping up': X-ray exposures in contemporary radiographic practice. *Radiography,* 22(2), pp. 194–198.

Hayre, C.M. Blackman, and S. Eyden, A. (2016b) Do general radiographic examinations resemble a person-centred environment? *Radiography,* 22(4), pp. e245–e251.

Hayre, C.M. Blackman, S. Carlton, K. and Eyden, A. (2019) The use of cropping and digital side markers (DSM) in digital radiography. *Journal of Medical Imaging and Radiation Sciences,* 50(2), pp. 234–242

Hayre, C.M. Blackman, S., Hackett, P.M.W., Muller, D., and Sim, J. Ethnography and medicine: The utility of positivist methods in ethnographic research. *Anthropology and Medicine.* (In Press). https://doi.org/10.1080/13648470.2021.1893657

Hayre, C.M. Jeffery, C., and Bungay, H. (2020) Do lead-rubber aprons always limit ionising radiation to radiosensitive organs? *Radiography.* 26(4), pp. e264–e269

Hayre, C.M. Bungay, H., Jeffery, C., Cobb, C. and Atutornu, J. (2018a) Can placing lead-rubber inferolateral to the light beam diaphragm limit ionising radiation to multiple radiosensitive organs? *Radiography.* 24(1), pp.15–21.

Holkup, PA., Tripp-Reimer, T., Salois, EM., and Weinert, C. (2004) Community-based participatory research – an approach to intervention research with a native American community. *ANS Advance Nurse Science.* 27(3), pp.162–175.

Howard, N. (2016) An open letter to *The BMJ* editors on qualitative research. *BMJ,* 352, p. i563.

Husain, S.T., Lei, S., Akram, T., Haider, M.J., Hussain, S.H., and Ali, M. (2018) Kurt Lewin's change model: A critical review of the role of leadership and employee involvement in organizational change. *Journal of Innovation & Knowledge.* 3(3), pp.123–127.

Husserl, E. (2010) *The Idea of Phenomenology.* Springer.

Kada, S., Satinovic, M., Booth, L., and Miller, P.K. (2018) Managing discomfort and developing participation in non-emergency MRI: Children's coping strategies during their first procedure. *Radiography.* 25 (1), pp.10–15.

Koopman, O. (2015) Phenomenology as a potential methodology for subjective knowing in science education research. *Indo-Pacific Journal of Phenomenology.* 15(1), pp.1–10.

Larsson W, Aspelin M, Bergquist K, Hillergard B, and Jacobsson L. (2007) The effects of PACS on radiographers work practice. *Radiography.* 13(3): pp. 235–240.

Laverty, SM. (2003) *Hermeneutic phenomenology and phenomenology: A comparison of historical and methodological considerations. International Institute for Qualitative Methodology.* 2(3), pp.21–35.

Lewin, K (1946) Action research and minority problems. *Journal of Sociology.* 2(4), pp. 34–46.

Lundvall, L., Dahlgre, M.A., and Wirell, S. (2014) Professionals' experiences of imaging in the radiography process – A phenomenological approach. *Radiography.* 20(1), pp. 48–52.

MacDonald, C. (2012) Understanding participatory action research: A qualitative research methodology option. *Canadian Journal of Action Research.* 13 (2), pp. 34–50.

Malinowski, B. (1984) *Argonauts of the Western Pacific.* Waveland Press.

Mercado, L and Hayre, C.M. (2018) The detection of wooden foreign bodies: An experimental study comparing direct digital radiography (DDR) and ultrasonography. *Radiography*. 24 (3), pp. 340–344.

Murphy, F., Nightingale, J., Hogg, P., Robinson, L., Seddon, D., and MacKay, S. (2015) Compression fore behaviours: An exploration of the beliefs and values influencing the application of breast compression during screening mammography. *Radiography*. 21 (1), pp. 30–35.

Naylor, S. and Foulkes, D. (2018) Diagnostic radiographers working in the operating theatre: An action research project. *Radiography*. 24(1), pp. 9–14.

Nichols, N., Griffith, A., and McLarnon, M. (2017) Community-based and participatory approaches in institutional ethnography. *Perspectives On and From institutional Ethnography Studies in Qualitative Methodology*. 15(1), pp. 107–124.

Nightingale, J.M., Murphy, F., Eaton, C., and Borgen, R. (2016). A qualitative analysis of staff-client interactions within a breast cancer assessment clinic. *Radiography*. 23(1): pp. 38–47.

Praag, L.V., Stevens, P.A.J., and Houtte, M.V. (2017) How humor makes or breaks student-teacher relationships: A classroom ethnography in Belgium. *Teaching and Teacher Education*. 66, pp. 393–401.

Rennie, D.L. (1998) Grounded theory methodology – The pressing need for a coherent logic of justification. *Theory & Psychology*. 8(1), pp. 101–119.

Sevens, T.J. and Reeves, P.J. (2019) Professional protectionism: A barrier to employing a sonographer graduate. *Radiography*. 25(1), pp. 77–82.

Snaith, B (2016) Evidence based radiography: Is it happening or are we experiencing practice creep and practice drift? *Radiography*. 22 (1), pp. 267–268.

Strauss, AL. (1987) *Qualitative Analysis for Social Scientists*. Cambridge, UK:Cambridge University Press.

Tie, YC., Birks, M., and Francis, K. (2019) Grounded theory research: A design framework for novice researchers. *Sage Open Medicine*. 7(1), pp. 1–8

Udas, K (1998) Participatory action research as critical pedagogy. *Systemic Practice and Action Research*. 11(6), pp. 599–628

Walsh, NA. (2010) Grounded theory for radiotherapy practitioners: Informing clinical practice. *Radiography*. 16 (3), pp. 244–247.

Strauss, A., Schatzman, D., Ehrlich, R., Bucher, M., and Sabshin, C. (1963) The hospital and its negotiated order. In: Friedson, E., ed. *The Hospital in Modern Society*. New York: Free Press, pp. 147–169.

Strudwick, R. The radiographic image: A cultural artefact? *Radiography*. 20(2), pp. 143–147.

The, A.M., Hak, T., Koeter, G., de Wal, G.V. (2000) Collusion in doctor-patient communication about imminent death: an ethnographic study. *BMJ*. 321, pp. 1376–1381.

Vindrola-Padros, C (2021). *Rapid Ethnographies – A Practical Guide*. Cambridge, UK: Cambridge University Press.

9 Data Collection in Qualitative Research

Christopher M. Hayre

9.1 INTRODUCTION

In this chapter, the focus is on qualitative methods, coupled with methodological considerations for qualitative researchers as they remain key during any data collection process. This chapter begins by discussing how ethical and moral boundaries in the field influence decision-making and research practice. This is important due to the exploratory nature of qualitative research and thus requires action or inaction in certain circumstances. Then, three central and commonly used methods will be detailed in order to not only provide insight into differences but also draw from experience. Other methodological considerations and questions surrounding 'where and when' it is ok to collect data, coupled with recognizing virtues associated with researcher positionality and reflexivity. It is anticipated that radiography students and early career researchers will find these insights helpful, not only theoretically but also from a practical standpoint following the application of such methods both within and outside of radiography.

9.2 ESTABLISHING ETHICAL AND MORAL BOUNDARIES

It is important to understand the role of qualitative research. Unlike quantitative research whereby the researcher seeks to remain at a distance when collecting data via survey or, say, experimentation. This section seeks to reflect on the process of qualitative data collection whilst providing some insight into practical approaches. By recognizing the role and practice of qualitative research in the natural setting it determines data generation strategies and perhaps importantly, greater acceptance and utility. Chapter 4 recognized the role of research ethics, as a general principle and how it is central to understand and prepare ethical applications upon seeking human participation. However, little is written about the ethical and moral considerations researchers face whilst in the field in radiography research. This is by no means a one size fits all outlook, as we have already come to appreciate. Instead, many constructions and perceptions can be accepted beyond the scope of this chapter. The nature of qualitative research and interconnection with the researcher is individually crafted (Denzin, 1997), yet experiences outlined here may help with certain

DOI: 10.1201/9780367559311-9

decision-making amongst future researchers. The establishment of moral and ethical boundaries prior to embarking in the field remains critical. For instance, prior to entering the hospital environment in the author's own work, it was decided that if any criminal activity (whilst highly unlikely) were observed, it would be reported, both within and outside of the radiography department (Hayre, 2016). Further, decisions to report unprofessional practice, such as aggressive behaviour, albeit from practitioners or patients would also be reported (ibid). Thankfully, neither of the abovementioned were observed; however, there are other considerations worthy of discussion, which are important to reflect upon here.

During my observations using an ethnographic methodology, it was decided not to involve paediatric patients. Whilst a critical area of practice, the imaging of children or infants can often be a traumatic experience for children undergoing radiographic examinations (Alexander, 2012); thus, it was felt that my presence may further hinder or heighten an already distressing situation. In addition, the research questions posed in my PhD were not specifically focused in paediatric imaging, thus remained an area of practice that could be omitted. On occasions whereby a radiographer entered the X-ray room to begin a paediatric examination I would exit the room in response to these duties. Looking back, whilst this remained an ethical consideration prior to the research commencing, it is clearly an area whereby an ethical and moral 'line' was drawn, based on my own predispositions as a diagnostic radiographer.

In clinical situations whereby my role as a radiographer and researcher became 'blurred' are reflected in scenarios when intervention was needed (Hayre et al., 2017). Earlier in chapter 4, my reflections of intervention were necessary to prevent unnecessary X-ray exposure to patients and also centred on questions from participants questioning their radiographic technique. The latter would vary as radiographers asked about preferred exposure settings, supported with questions pertaining to positioning for certain examinations (Hayre, 2016). This naturally identifies intervening in situations that should be observed in its 'natural state'. Upon offering a professional opinion to participants, it arguably impeded any natural development to radiographic practices or behaviours from some radiographers. Methodologically, however, the assistance provided to radiographers (especially junior radiographers) offered advantages. For instance, assisting radiographers with questions or suggestions helped build rapport with the participant(s). Being helpful and approachable as a researcher in the X-ray environment later supported invitations to interviews and ongoing engagement with observational methods. This example highlights two important features. First, whilst my primary role remained a researcher, it was difficult to wholly distance myself as a registered radiographer, demonstrating opposing duties, a duty to engage and assist with colleagues in a similar way to a senior radiographer, coupled with seeking to capture naturally occurring phenomena. Second, the establishment of ethical and moral boundaries prior to moving into the research field may lead to occasions or situations in the clinical environment that require researchers to assist, when applicable. The unpredictable nature of hospital settings naturally offers some uncertainly around 'where' and 'when' assistance may take place; however, our ethical and moral duties as healthcare professionals should also take precedent in light of facilitating the healthcare setting.

Another example resides in the decision-making to socialize with members at a particular research site. Having worked in the clinical context, as a locum radiographer, as well as observe and interview participants as a researcher, this naturally led to the forming of social circles. Although technically in the role as a researcher and ethnographer, a decision was made to join colleagues/participants on 'evening drinks' and accept an invitation to the Christmas party (Hayre, 2016). Looking back, was this overstepping the moral and ethical duties as an ethnographer whereby I became 'too close' with participants, perhaps 'going native'? The counter-argument and one that remains advocated here is former social encounters co-existing with professional and personal interactions in the field. Furthermore, as rapport building continued, this not only indirectly facilitated relationships with participants, it naturally helped immersion within the culture, albeit existential to the research environment itself. In my view, this form of 'blurring' of ethical and moral boundaries is important to recognize as qualitative researchers and especially in scenarios where research resides in the natural setting. In short, whilst researchers may find themselves conflicting with their role and engagements to social events, the positives to such events can help build rapport, which may lead to richer empirical data.

9.3   DATA COLLECTION METHODS

9.3.1   OBSERVATIONS

Observations in qualitative research are an important tool for data collection. This method requires a researcher to become the key instrument, using his/her senses to capture the social world around them. Simply put, everything, whether seen, heard, smelt or felt can be recorded as 'data' (Burgess, 1993). Observation remains an integral part of healthcare practice and role of the radiographer. Notably, radiographers begin their radiographic examinations by observing their patients, ascertaining ambulatory state, consciousness and/or ability to undergo the examination itself. Thus, the practice of observing our everyday space as radiographers can be attributed to the same value in terms of empirical research. Barley (1986, p.83) in his early observations of computed tomography acknowledged that in order to identify patterns and practice behaviour requires reliance on observation to record interactions. In my own work, the observational method not only offered a tool for data collection but also enabled the ability to 'get closer' to participants in order to build trust and openness with members of the team (Hammersley, 1992). This allowed participants to become familiar with the researcher's intentions, coincided with the goals of the research project.

There are three accepted observational strategies whereby a researcher remains overt. First, the 'observer as participant' enables a researcher to strive towards being immersed within a particular group or sub-group of people (Pole and Morrison, 2003). For cultural studies, this will involve prolonged engagement with participants in order to acquire some 'insider' knowledge of that particular group and remains the primary role as an ethnographer (Rudge, 1995). Second, a 'participant as observer' differs as the researcher becomes engaged with participants but is still regarded as a researcher (Sheppard, 2007). There were occasions from experience that transcended into this position, depending on participants observed, the clinical examination taking place and/or the need for intervention, as outlined earlier. Third, the complete observer is an approach to observation whereby the researcher wholly distances themselves from the participants. The 'complete observer' remains overt and at a distance from his/her participant(s) (ibid) and may involve an 'outsider perspective', such as a social anthropologist observing medical imaging examinations. Their 'participation' would not be necessary, practical or even ethical as they are not healthcare professionals. In short, the complete observer seeks to merely observe and have no interaction with the participants or setting under observation (Pole and Morrison, 2003).

For a researcher seeking to perform covert research, this is usually referred to as 'complete participation'. In this situation, the researcher decides to be fully embedded in the research setting, like a spy (Johnson, 2018). In radiography, this would involve the researcher being, say, employed as a radiographer or a radiography assistant to hide their true identity, but permitted to enter the X-ray room. For covertness, participants will be unaware they are being observed during their clinical work. It is often referenced as 'going native', as alluded in indigenous fieldwork, for instance, and also remains commonplace in other texts (Hammersley and Atkinson, 2007). The type of observation will depend on the research questions and length of study, but perhaps more importantly, it needs to be identified and later critiqued for ethical appropriateness.

During observations, it is important to collect as much information as possible, but this will vary depending on the abovementioned strategy. From experience, the use of an A5 notebook helped 'jot down' notes and make comments. However, this may not always be appropriate. Upon observing suboptimum radiographic practices, it was not always appropriate to document specific information in order to prevent rebuttals with participants. Further, as observations progressed, it was important to alter notetaking practices by using shorthand symbols, representing actions by radiographers. Examples included the action of 'cropping' or non-adjustment of X-ray exposures, improper use of the source to image distance (SID), and so forth, often denoted by shapes. On reflection, as observations progressed, notetaking also developed to capture the right information and within an appropriate timeframe. On rare occasions, it was necessary to 'ditch' my notebook in response to an immediate sense of hostility (Hayre and Hackett, 2020). On this occasion, it was felt that taking handwritten notes would only heighten the sensitivity of my presence in the field. In order to capture some observations, it was often necessary to 'dash' to the toilet and record notes via a Dictaphone (ibid). This experience has been reported elsewhere (Burgess, 1990) and demonstrates that whilst notetaking remains a common tool and widely appreciated in overt research, there are situations where alternate forms of data collection are needed in order to prevent additional barriers or disengagement with participants.

9.3.2 INTERVIEWS

Interviews remain a critical method in qualitative research and are used across most qualitative research designs. Interviews can be divided into three categories: structured, semi-structured or unstructured and typically performed on a one-to-one basis with the researcher and participant. This provides an alternate way of gathering insightful data concerning a particular topic. Interviews are useful because they allow researchers to ask questions to a participant that remains away from the gaze of others. This is useful because if a question was posed to an individual in the X-ray viewing room or in a focus group, for instance, the answer may be crafted or shaped in order to resonate with peers. Throughout the interview process, participants are likely to provide open and honest responses knowing their commentary remains strictly anonymous. The type of interview, however, will not only determine the dialogue between researcher and participant but also determine the potential for elaboration or alternate discussion. For example, structured interviews contain a set of questions offering little deviation. Similar to survey questions, there is limited room for discussion amongst the researcher and participant and thus may lack 'depth'. Semi-structured interviews offer more flexibility in terms of delivery because although the researcher has a set of preformatted questions, based on existing knowledge or previous methods (quantitative or qualitative), there are opportunities for the participant (or researcher) to diverge, expand and discuss ideas that reasonate with both participant and researcher. Lastly, unstructured interviews oppose structure by negating preconceived questions by the researcher. They often omit an interview schedule, often used to keep the researcher on track with his or her questioning. Whilst these will contain 'depth', they may lack focus, leading to unasked questions. These types of interviews are performed when little is known about a topic or used as an initial method to generate theory concerning a particular phenomenon or concept.

Interviews allow for the exploration of attitudes, beliefs and behaviours of key members and are undertaken to provide deeper meaning as to why they act in a certain way, for instance. Further, whilst observations may capture optimum and suboptimum practices amongst radiographers, it may be important to understand why this behaviour has occurred. In addition, being aware of 'sensitive practices' amongst radiographers, such as the selection of X-ray exposures, use of lead-rubber for radiation protection, coupled with knowledge and understanding of image acquisition. In short, the use of semi-structured interviewing not only 'builds' on from observations made, but also provides a 'controlled space' to ask sensitive questions, away from the cultural group. This can naturally provide unique and rich responses, which are later supported with observational, or perhaps survey data. If deciding whether a structured or semi-structured is best appropriate, it is important to consider the type of questioning and current understanding of the topic at hand. It is also generally accepted that in order to provide 'good interview questions', it requires open-ended questioning. A closed question, for instance, would only allow a participant to answer 'yes' or 'no', such as: 'Do you use X-ray exposures appropriately in practice? However, an example of an open-ended question may read: Can you tell me your experiences with X-ray exposures and how you apply these in practice? Here, the open-ended question seeks to draw on the experiences of participants with supporting clinical application. In my own research, the utilization of observations enhances questions, drawing on 'what had been seen' in being able to generate some theoretical underpinnings for future questioning, such as: 'Upon my observations of X-ray exposures I noticed that radiographers rarely manipulated the pre-set exposures on the X-ray console. What are your experiences with X-ray exposure manipulation?' Here, the rationale for little exposure manipulation is reinforced by previous observations, asserting some empirical validity in this method, which is argued to obtain a better response. The examples above seek to enrich the time spent with participants, whilst attempting to provide greater insight and depth from the interview method.

Sampling is an important feature when selecting participants for interviews. It is important for researchers to select participants that are willing to continue their engagement with the study (if applicable), but also those deemed appropriate. Initial thoughts perhaps challenge how many interviews are required in order to capture and answer research questions. Whilst no prescribed number is documented in light of the explorative inquiry, my own 'knee jerk' reaction was to perform as many as possible, as it would somehow seem 'better'. Looking back, upon finishing interviewing, there was always the desire to just take one more interview and postpone forthcoming analytical processes. Importantly, however, for prospective researchers, it is recommended that interviews are ceased upon reaching data saturation – the time in which all research questions have been satisfactorily answered. Ceasing interviews requires confidence in order to ensure no further information is necessary, which is driven by initial research questions.

The time taken to conduct an interview may also vary and will depend on interactions and responses with participants. From experience, semi-structured interviews vary between 15 and 60 minutes, but can also exceed this. It is important not to rush participants, especially within the semi-structured style of questioning. Upon listening back on initial interview recordings I would often 'speak over' the participant. These interruptions would break the narrative and prove problematic when transcribing. Further, it is important to allow participants to think, and whilst this may result in a period of silence when recording, it can help participants' recollect reactions, attitudes and/or behaviours. On the other hand, it may be evident that participants seek a conclusion, and thus important to try and maintain and sense of time for participants in order to reaffirm their interest. This is rare, but acknowledged during fieldwork and also important to ensure participants are not uncomfortable if time expectations are exceeded.

Capturing interview data is clearly paramount and usually performed using a digital audio device. There are a number of methods that facilitate this with the use of smartphones or Dictaphones. The latter is recommended because it usually offers longer battery life when compared to smart devices. The use of a smart mobile device can be useful as a backup device, in case of technical difficulties or malfunctions with Dictaphones. The place of the interview is also an important feature. Interviews should be conducted in a quiet environment, with little background noise. Some Dictaphones offer enhanced sensitivity thus likely to detect background noise if building work, or conversations with staff are taking place, which may also lead to difficulties transcribing interviews. If encountering an environment that has background noise, it is important to 'playback' any initial recordings to assess the quality and ascertain whether the interview location should be changed.

As part of the interview process, it is not uncommon for qualitative researchers to develop topics or add themes to their interview schedule. For example, a common practice for most qualitative interviewers offers a penultimate question: Is there anything else in this interview you would like to discuss, perhaps something I have failed to mention? This question is critical for two reasons. First, not only does it offer the participant an opportunity to discuss a topic of their choosing, in response to the interview being developed from the researcher's interpretation, experience and assumptions. Second, the question and any subsequent responses allows the researcher to potentially incorporate other questions previously underexplored with follow-up interviewees. In short, whilst participants provide insightful empirical feedback concerning values, beliefs, opinions and attitudes towards certain events, they can assist with the methodological development of the schedule. By recognizing the valued input of participants we are able to provide depth and substance to the overall research and generate themes as the research progresses.

9.3.3 FOCUS GROUPS

Focus groups are an important method in qualitative research. Whilst generally similar to interviews, whereby a researcher (or other mediator) asks pertinent questions, they instead involve multiple participants. A key advantage of most focus groups is the gathering of perspectives, beliefs and attitudes from participants within a single environment. The focus group is not simply asking the same question to all participants, but to generate discussion amongst the participants. This allows an exchange of ideas amongst individuals, which may differ, allowing the researcher to explore other points of view. The number of participants in each focus group can vary depending on the topic but typically ranges from 3–21 (circa 10 participants) (Nyumba et al., 2018). In my own experience, it will depend on the topic and availability of participants. This type of method has been found useful in an array of academic disciplines. For example, in business, the use of focus groups is often used to assess consumables in order to ascertain certain products prior to being sold on the open market (Calder, 1977). In politics, focus groups are used during election campaigns in order to ascertain certain policies or impressions of party leaders (Stanley, 2016). Whilst originally used for film and television, focus groups also examine educational messages from governments regarding a particular illness or health behaviour (Wilkinson, 1998). At a discipline-based level, for radiography, focus groups have uncovered the radiographer's role in child protection (Davis and Reeves, 2006), the care for dementia patients in medical imaging and the role of MRI radiographers towards patient care (Challen, Low and McEntee, 2018).

Focus groups offer a unique way of approaching a research topic. For instance, the nature of bringing a cohort of participants together allows the emergence of opinions pertaining to a particular theme, such as exploring academic assessment feedback amongst student radiographers. The application of focus groups can capitalize on differing perspectives, which from experience stimulate different debates. Interestingly and throughout such discussions, it is important for mediators to allow discussions to evolve and offer prompts, when appropriate, to seek clarification on opposing or supporting statements. Whilst healthy discussion and debate are good, there is a caveat that can lead to individuals being suppressed by stronger characters or personalities. Examples where overpowering discussions or narratives are intended to suppress voices and opinions of others requires alternate tactics with the mediator by subconsciously identifying the suppression and then finding a way to draw out the opinions of others.

Data collection techniques for focus groups range from audio recording, note-taking and participant observation (Stewart, Shamdasani and Rook, 2007). Data collection methods are important to consider because if an audio device is used alone, it may be difficult to discern voices (if participant labels are required). Further, during a topical issue, some participants may talk over one another, which becomes problematic for transcription. Here, it is the role of the mediator to ensure that individuals are heard but also not spoken over. One way of achieving this is by asking participants to raise their hand if wishing to speak, providing a sign to the mediator that he/she would like to offer his or her opinion. In addition, as a medi-ator of focus groups in a study involving people with dementia, it was decided that two mediators remain present. This was invaluable as the second mediator offered an 'insiders perspective' for participants (Hayre, Tyrrell and Strudwick, 2018). She was not only able to observe non-verbal cues and interactions with participants, but also resonate with participants on a personal level. This demonstrates that whilst one mediator may be focused on asking research questions and actively listen to participants' responses, other conversations may naturally develop amongst the participants, which were also valuable. This experience demonstrates that where applicable, more than one mediator can facilitate data collection by using a variety of data collection tools in order to enhance the interactions between participants and the mediators themselves.

The role of a mediator is also important to reflect upon. The abovementioned example highlights the importance that participants are not consciously or uncon-sciously led into false responses. Examples in the literature highlight how participants have altered their behaviour in order to prevent others from criticizing staff in a long-term residential care home (Kitzinger, 1995). Clearly, for focus groups, this remains a limitation whereby participants from the same cohort are identifiable to one another, which, in turn, could lead to dismay amongst peers. Further, there is also the pos-sibility that such outspokenness is not kept confidential outside the focus group, which may have repercussions for the participant (ibid). Whilst unlikely, the role of focus group often plays a pivotal role by liberating those by providing 'a voice'. The study concerning people with dementia not only provided empirical evidence but also facilitated group cohesion (Hayre, Tyrrell and Strudwick, 2018). In this study, the purpose, whilst evaluative, indirectly brought individuals together via some 'social togetherness' (ibid). This unexpected outcome, from experience, was valuable to individuals allowing people with dementia to simply sit and talk to peers living with a similar condition, which was later enhanced with refreshments. In short, the focus group had a positive, yet unintentional social role. This supports the notion that whilst focus groups are typically used by researchers to explore a number of in-depth perspectives for empirical gain, it may also act as a therapeutic tool, methodologic-ally, whereby individuals share experiences, leading to self-development, or perhaps, friendships. Looking back, informal discussions with the participants were not only recognized by the Dementia Service but also offered social benefits brought out by the research process itself.

For sampling, the number of focus groups that may take place will vary. Similarly with interviewing, participants are purposively sampled, following consent, in order to try and capture the views of those experiencing the phenomena first-hand. Clearly, for people with dementia, a fine balance is required to ask those who were able to participate with respect to cognitive health. Here, purposive sampling not only focused on persons with dementia but also selected participants who would be able to take part (Hayre, Tyrrell and Strudwick, 2018). This was achieved using closely affiliated care workers who cared for those living with dementia in the community in order to ensure individuals were able to undergo questioning (ibid). The associated advantages of focus groups allow researchers to capture a number of different perspectives within a single event. This can provide a unique lens into a culture, phenomena or service being studied. It also offers a sound platform for ascertaining both supporting and conflicting perspectives, whereby attitudes and behaviours are discussed amongst the group.

9.4   WHERE AND WHEN IS IT OK TO COLLECT DATA?

The thought of considering whether it is safe to collect data in the field may not immediately resonate with early career researchers. Obvious safety requirements concerning ionizing radiation, or the use of magnetic fields, for example, are pertinent hazards within our everyday work. Yet, other components such as researcher safety, sensitivity, and hostility should also be acknowledged, albeit rarely discussed within the qualitative space in radiography research. Fortunately, reports of hostile encounters between radiographers and patients are not commonplace (Lane, 2016). Hostile encounters are likely to occur inter-professionally in medical imaging between radiographers and radiologists (Ehrlich and Coakes, 2020, p.101). Looking back on ethnographic observations, although hostile situations were not commonplace, they did, on occasion, occur. To say that hostility [a showing or feeling of opposition or dislike] will not take place, nor exist, is misplaced. For those researchers thinking of engaging in the workspace as a means of empirical exploration, they must accept and document the possibility of hostile encounters during the fieldwork and how best to mitigate and manage if it occurs.

During data collection at one research site, there was an immediate sense of heightened sensitivity surrounding my PhD topic. For some participants, it led to comments such as '*are we passing for you?*' and/or '*are we doing well enough for you?*' (Hayre and Hackett, 2020, p.51). At the time, initial questions indicated sensitivity for participants upon observations of their practice. This is often termed the 'culture shock' whereby confrontation can arise with participants in observational research (Hammersley and Atkinson, 2007, p.91). Further, participants may also differ in their opinion of the researcher – some found the topic fascinating, whereas others failed to see its purpose. The key for most researchers is to remain balanced between identifying the appropriateness of collecting sensitive data via qualitative methods, with overcoming social awkwardness, which may later manifest in hostile behaviour (ibid). Little evidence exists discussing emotion or locality for sensitive or hostile situations in radiography. Whilst recognized in the field of sociology, whereby methodologically, it enhances the trustworthiness of a study (Blackman, 2007), there is perhaps an unspoken reticence in exploring emotion and locality between the researcher and research environment in radiography (ibid), leading to what is simply an underrepresentation in the literature. In the work of Blackman (2007), this subtle but important consideration can be attributed to what is known as 'hidden eth-nography' whereby critical, sensitive or hostile encounters remain 'hidden' from the reader. The rationale for suppressing emotional events is often suggestive of empir-ical usefulness. For example, Barter and Renold (2003, p.100) assert that emotion in research is considered 'epistemologically irrelevant'. Coffey (1999) also warns us that younger academics are less likely to provide realistic accounts, as they, themselves, try to build and sustain academic careers, seeking 'acceptance' within their com-munity. Clearly, the notion of simply accepting or writing about sensitive and hos-tile encounters may become an immediate deterrent for budding academics in their careers. In my own view, experiences of hostile situations (see Hayre and Hackett, 2020, p.47) in multi-sited fieldwork initially led to the feeling of disappointment. Yet, after leaving the field, followed by discussions with peers and reflection over a period of time, the incident naturally enhances my own methodological evaluations as a researcher during fieldwork. Fortunately, engagement with research sites prior to this encounter was not commonplace. The spectrum of feeling welcomed by some or alienation by others later appreciated a 'multi-sited research imaginary', critically evaluating the multi-sited approach (Hayre and Hackett (2020, p. 49). Abu-Lughod (2000, p. 264) supports this reasoning whereby partaking in multi-sited research can draw on methodological comparisons that seek to understand our emotion and locality, whilst engaging with power structures within.

Fielding (2011, p. 249) recognizes hostility as a situation whereby a research sample remains actively resistant to research, leading to implications around access to the research environment or data itself. Further, Fielding (2011) adds that it may not be the researcher *per se* that defines the problem, but the questions or answers he or she seeks to uncover. Whilst this latter assertion is noted, leading to hostile events, the 'physical position' within the research space, in my view, also facilitated intru-sion and invasiveness for some participants in the field, which is believed to have supported the abovementioned experience (Hayre and Hackett, 2020). In short, for prospective researchers utilizing qualitative methods such as participant observation, interviews or focus groups, it is sensible to try and foresee sensitive questioning or topics that may be threatening to research participants. From experience, deciding to leave the research field, agreed by the gatekeeper at the time, demonstrates the unpredictable nature of qualitative inquiry in radiographic research. Whilst impos-sible to fully predict any outcome or decision if/when it occurs, it is critical that both researcher positionality and reflexivity are engaged, which is now discussed.

9.5 RESEARCHER POSITIONALITY AND REFLEXIVITY

For qualitative researchers, their positional and reflexive attributes remain intertwined in the research process and thus important to report. The positionality and reflexive actions of the researcher arguably take place the moment (s)he enters the field. Efforts to identify our positionality begins by introducing ourselves. For example, I would describe myself as a diagnostic radiographer, born, raised and educated in the United Kingdom, who (at the time of writing this book) resides in Australia. I would then think about my interests, both practically and from a research perspective, perhaps my rationale for writing this book and desire to move into education. A self-positional statement seeks to unravel who the researcher is now, and what impact they are likely to have during the research process. Positionality is concerned with outlining individual views on the world and positions adopted about a research topic. In chapter 2, the term 'ontology' is used to discern the perspective [as outsiders or readers] in order 'see where the researcher is coming from'. It enables readers to understand how the researcher is viewing a particular phenomenon from their position. Central to this reflect our values and beliefs, which may drive our undertaking of research in the first place. In my own doctoral study, it began by identifying me as a researcher, chapter 1 (Hayre, 2016). Here discussions concerning family and illness, and experiences of education in childhood through to higher education, coupled with observations as a radiography student and radiographer. Upon reflection, these features help develop 'who I was' and to some degree, and at this point in time, the development of my thesis.

There are, of course, other personal characteristics that are either culturally or generally ascribed. For instance, as a white heterosexual male, from the United Kingdom, these are personal characteristics that remain both historical and contemporary. For example, what impact would my current characteristics have upon deciding to perform a similar study to Malinowski in 1922 with Aboriginal Australian communities? Our positionality is not simply about how we engage with research participants and the environment around us, it also questions how participants and communities engage with us. As a native British Citizen temporarily residing in Australia at the time of writing this book, I recollect upon a recently commissioned edited book with colleagues in the United Kingdom and the United States of America. This book aims to explore the use of digital technology in qualitative research. My co-editors and I decided to seek contributions from our respective indigenous communities in the United States and Australia, respectively. However, our requests to known researchers in the field failed to reciprocate a response. Upon reconvening, as editors, and later reflecting, we wondered whether as four white editors, three males and one female, our request was perhaps regarded as discourteous or somehow offensive. Whilst not intentional, it is possible that our topic could have been regarded as sensitive and perhaps unjust. Could historical attributes of both imperialism and colonialism provide a rationale for this enhanced sensitivity? In Australia for example, the view of imperialism and colonialism is best observed by 'Australia Day', a public holiday celebrated on the 26th January each year. Whilst a day, for some, celebratory marking the anniversary of the 1788 arrival of the First Fleet at Port Jackson in New South Wales, it is also regarded as 'Invasion Day' and/or 'National Day of Mourning' by some Indigenous Australians and others sympathetic to the cause. Here, we observe a counter-celebration with arguments that it should be abolished entirely. The point here is that as individuals we may bring our own history, culture and values that may not be agreeable with others, and whilst they may hold egalitarian motives within the society, our unconscious intentions may still remain insensitive.

Importantly, then, in order for us to respect the practices, culture and history of others, we should seek to examine our own positionality in the research space, as we do in our everyday society. This is typically regarded as 'otherness' and seen to be valuable for researchers examining intercultural research (Guttormsen, 2018). This sense of 'otherness' is not dissimilar from our role as diagnostic radiographers. Radiographers transnationally interact and communicate with a range of cultures different from their own. Remaining sensitive, then, to alternate perspectives and beliefs is generally recognized, and whilst this readily takes place in our practice setting, we should remain mindful in our research settings. As we attempt to foreground our positionality in order to help evade inherent weaknesses, there are natural elements we cannot fully forgo in order to omit perceptions others may have.

The overall narrative of this textbook demonstrates positionality to readers within individual chapters. For instance, discussions of hostile encounters or necessary intervention are deeply acknowledged. These are positional characteristics because it is who I am, both a radiographer and individual, which naturally led to such scenarios. If imagining for a moment that observations were from a sociologist standpoint, not radiographic, then notably the above experiences may have differed, in light of different experiences and/or expertise. Further, our positionality is reaffirmed in terms of how participants view us via our connection with inherent perspectives, but also the researcher's apparent disassociation, whereby discussions with participants lead to unconventional questions: *'why on earth did you decide to do that'* and *'what do you intend to do after it?'*. On the one hand, this facilitates the social poise of 'friend' with 'familiarity', later facilitating radiographers with questions or prevention of X-ray exposures. On the other hand, my eagerness to embark on a PhD close after graduation provided an association as the 'stranger', intellectually and socially, thus distancing myself from peers (Hammersley and Atkinson, 2007, p. 100). The role of positionality, then, is not simply how we reflect on our status characteristics and experiences in order to become 'socially aware' of our impact, it also appreciates how individuals' behave and react to prior thoughts and feelings. Whilst we cannot comprehend the thought processes of others, their actions or inactions may offer further opportunities for evaluation as we make our way through the research process.

Reflexivity, in addition to positionality, is interlinked and naturally coexists in order to engage the researcher in critical reflections prior, during and post research. Researchers involved in qualitative research designs often have a myriad of responsibilities to themselves, their participants, and the overarching goals of the research. These inevitably influence the practice, interpretation and prospective dissemination of qualitative data. Being 'reflexive' enables readers of qualitative studies to build 'trust' with his/her readership via open and honest events taking place, and as research progresses (Adams, 2004). It also allows the researcher to not only acknowledge his/her actions and behaviours in the research environment but to 'open up' and disclose interactions, reactions and influences had. Reflexive thinking and actions take place from the moment the researcher enters the research environment; interactions with gatekeepers, the consensual processes, initial data collection, data collection tools and ways of managing expectations or queries from participants. Again, the practice of reflexivity is not simply prescribed in the sub-section of this chapter but integrated throughout. It cannot be considered as a 'box-ticking exercise' to satisfy the qualitative framework, which is readily recognizable. Instead, it requires critical engagement with self and how such actions have influenced topic selection, method selection, participant engagement and analysis of data in radiography research in order to provide deeper contextual meaning to the research context.

In my own experience, the use of reflexivity helped shape a number of concerns emerging early in the research process. One example resides in the collection of data during observational methods. For example, prior to entering the clinical environment, it was felt necessary to design a 'precise' data sheet that would collect detailed parameters of radiographic examinations. Parameters such as kVp, mAs, source to image distance (SID), filtration, and field size were considered important and essential for each examination (Hayre, 2016). However, after several minutes of observation, it was obvious that this predetermined method of data collection was not only intrusive but prevented radiographers from performing radiographic examinations in a timely manner, especially during busy periods (ibid). In order to ensure it did not hinder the everyday and 'natural practice' of radiography, the A4 data collection sheet was discarded and replaced with an A5 notebook. This required 'reflexive actions' whereby the need for critical evaluation and application would help prevent added discomfort, distress or delay during radiographic examinations.

For new researchers engaging or reading about reflexivity for the first time, it is acknowledged that our reflexive actions are driven by our values (Greenbank, 2003). Positionality and reflexivity are important to demonstrate in our work because the nature of qualitative work may change, depending on the context, situation or individuals involved. Further, although positionality is helpful in contextualizing immediate values, beliefs and characteristics of the researcher, the utility of reflexivity helps inform or reform our positionality as a study progresses. Reflexivity is not about accepting weaknesses of subjectivity in radiographic research, but how to best overcome inherent interactions whilst delving deeper into social events. In my view, research positionality and reflexivity seek to enhance methodological honesty and robustness in qualitative research. Failing to acknowledge reflexive decision-making arguably fails to recognize the methodological design, which has ultimately lead to the generation of data.

9.6 CHAPTER SUMMARY

In this chapter, the focus has been to expand on data collection aspects in qualitative research. The chapter began by recognizing, how, as researchers, we are guided by ethical and moral boundaries when engaging with gatekeepers, participants and collecting fieldwork. The use of observations, interviews and focus groups as key methods have been identified, drawing from personal research experiences. Here, recognition of methodological considerations from within the literature and also those specific to radiography are provided to offer relevance to the radiography community. Other issues such as 'where and when' it may be safe to collect data, coincided with outlining reflexivity and positionality are identified. These remain important for researchers engaged in the qualitative space because above all else, the researcher remains a critical figure. Importantly, whilst opportunity will arise through original empiricism (the goal of any research), there may also be conflict and challenges to consider. Here, reflexivity remains pivotal as we navigate research encounters as researchers themselves weave through unknown possibilities. The journey of any qualitative researcher during data collection is not simply an opportunity by adding empirical evidence but also an opportunity for professional and personal development, methodologically.

KEY TERMS

Audio recording: is typically a technique used to record the audio sound of participants and/or the researcher during observations, interviews and/or focus groups.

Closed question: refers to a question whereby the participant either provides a simple yes or no answer, with little elaboration or is only able to provide a phase or word to a particular question.

Cohort: is regarded as a group of individuals who share a particular characteristic, for example, radiography students are considered a cohort in light of their shared characteristics with undertaking a radiography degree.

Complete observer: is a detached observer where the researcher is neither seen nor recognized by participants, i.e., via video cameras.

Complete participation: is a role in which a researcher is covertly placed in the research space. They may participate in the daily activities of the work, but also collect data without participants knowing.

Covert: is generally regarded as someone who is not openly acknowledging or displaying themselves.

Dictaphone: an audio device used to collect digital audio information.

Focus group: is similar to an interview, but will comprise more than one participant in order to enhance discussion and debate amongst participants.

Gatekeepers: are key members of the research fieldwork with which researchers make initial contact. They are typically associated with allowing access to the field and/or remaining a critical point of contact for researchers throughout the research.

Hidden ethnography: a concept that explores empirical data not previously published because it may be considered too controversial.

Hostility: to observe behaviour that is deemed unfriendly or in opposition.

Interview schedule: is a list containing either a structure or semi-structured set of questions that have been prepared by a researcher and used to help guide the interview process.

Mediator: is regarded as an impartial third party that can facilitate dialogue between members of a group.

Natural setting: is typically associated with qualitative research whereby researchers observe the everyday context under investigation.

Note-taking: is the practice of taking written, pictorial or audio notes within the research environment.

Observer as a participant: allows a researcher to participate in a group, yet the primary purpose is to collect data at a distance.

Open-ended questioning: is opposed to closed questions because they cannot be answered with a simple 'yes' or 'no'. Questions are phrased in a way that leads the participant to explain a situation or divulging about a particular experience.

Overt: is opposed to 'covert' and is performed or shown openly with those around them.

Participant as an observer: is where the research is known by the participants and regarded as more as a friend or colleague in the research space.

Positionality: seeks to identify the researcher by means of his/her values and status characteristics.

Prompts: is a term used during semi-structured or unstructured interviewing whereby researchers may ask an additional questions in order to prompt a 'richer' responses from the participant.

Reflexivity: is the ongoing process in which a researcher examines his/her own values actions and judgements throughout the research process. It is closely linked to positionality in order to critically reflect on what may occur in relation to individual positionality.

Sampling: is a process used in qualitative research that invites and selects participants pertinent to the study.

Transcription: is a process in which audio recordings are played back and typed accurately in order to represent the participant(s) voices.

Verbatim: refers to exactly the same words as were used originally and thus essential during the transcription process in order to capture words accurately.

EXERCISES AND STUDY QUESTIONS

1   If you are currently deciding which research methods to select, using the information above, list the advantages and disadvantages of each method and identify likely impact this will have on the empirical data uncovered.

2   When considering your data collection methods, it is important to establish your own ethical and moral boundaries. Think about potential incidences that may occur. Think about your own physical or virtual position. Upon identifying areas in which you think are inappropriate provide a short narrative asserting your response and approach to mitigate such events.

3   I recommend keeping a diary in order to capture your reflexivity and positional components during the research. If you are embarking on the research field, write about any preconceived ideas and be sure to critically evaluate your actions and reactions to any forthcoming occurrences that take place.

REFERENCES

Abu-Lughod, L. (2000) Locating ethnography. *Ethnography.* 1(1), pp. 261–267.

Adams, M. (2004) Whatever Will Be, Will Be: Trust, Fate and the Reflexive Self. *Culture & Psychology.* 10(4), pp. 387–408.

Alexander, M. (2012) Managing patient stress in pediatric radiology. *Radiologic Technology.* 83(6), pp. 549–560.

Johnson, M. (2018) Covert observation. In Allen, M. (Ed.) *The SAGE Encyclopedia of Communication Research Methods.* Thousand Oaks: Sage, pp. 286–289.

Barley, S.R. (1986) Technology as an occasion for structuring: Evidence from observations of CT scanners and the social order of radiology departments, *Administrative Science Quarterly,* 31(1), pp. 78–108.

Barton, C. and Reynold, E. (2003) Dilemmas of Control. In R. Lee and E. Stanko (eds.), *Researching Violence: Essays on Methodology and Measurement*. London: Routledge, pp. 88–106.

Blackman, S. (2007) 'Hidden ethnography': Crossing emotional boarders in qualitative accounts of young people's lives. *Sociology*. 41(4), pp. 699–716.

Burgess, R.G. (1990) *Studies in Qualitative Methodology – Reflections on Field Experience*. London: JAI press Inc.

Burgess, R.G. (1993) *In the Field: Introduction to Field Research*. New York: Routledge.

Calder, B. (1977) Focus groups and the nature of qualitative marketing research. *Journal of Marketing Research*. 14 (1), pp. 353–364.

Challen, R., Low, L.-F., and McEntee, M.F. (2018) Dementia patient care in the diagnostic medical imaging department. *Radiography*. 24 (1), pp. S33–S42.

Coffey, A. (1999) *The Ethnographic Self*. London: Sage.

Davis, M. and Reeves, P. (2006) The radiographer's role in child protection: Comparison of radiographers perceptions by use of focus groups. *Radiography*. 12(2), pp. 161–168.

Denzin, N. (1997) *Interpretive Ethnography*. London: Sage.

Ehrlich, R.A. and Coakes, D.M. 2020) *Patient Care in Radiography – With an Introduction to Medical Imaging*. (10th edn.). Elsiever: London.

Fielding, N. (2011) Working in Hostile Environments. In C. Seale, D. Silverman, J.F. Gumbrium and G. Gobo (eds.), *Qualitative Research in Practice*. Thousand Oaks, CA: Sage, p. 23.

Greenbank, P. (2003) The role of values in educational research: The case for reflexivity. *British Educational Research Journal*. 29(6), pp.791–801.

Guttormsen, D.S.A. (2018) Advancing otherness and othering of the cultural other during 'intercultural encounters' in cross-cultural management research. *International Studies of Management & Organsiation*. 48(3), pp. 314–332.

Hammersley, M. (1992) *What's Wrong With Ethnography*. New York: Routledge.

Hammersley, M. and Atkinson, P. (2007) *Ethnography Principles in Practice*. 3rd Ed. New York: Routledge.

Hayre, C.M. (2016) *Radiography observed: An ethnographic study exploring contemporary radiographic practice*. PhD Thesis. Canterbury Christ Church University. Faculty of Health and Wellbeing.

Hayre, C.M. Eyden, A. Blackman, S, and Carlton, K. (2017) Image acquisition in general radiography: The utilisation of DDR. *Radiography*. 23(2), pp. 147–152

Hayre, C.M. and Hackett, P.M.W. (2020) *Handbook of Ethnography in Healthcare Research*. New York: Routledge.

Hayre, C.M. Tyrrell, K. and Strudwick, R. (2018) Dementia Together Service – Updated: A mid-term evaluation of the Dementia Together Service by Sue Ryder, Ipswich, Suffolk. [Online] Available at: http://www.dementia-together.com/Content/Assets/Employer-Documents/DTMidTermEvaluation2018.pdf (Accessed: 30/03/2021).

Kitzinger, J. (1995) Qualitative research: Introducing focus groups. *BMJ*. *311*(299) doi: https://doi.org/10.1136/bmj.311.7000.299

Lane, A.N. (2016) Medical imaging and consent: When is an X-ray assault? *Journal of Medical Radiation Sciences*. 63(2), pp. 133–137.

Nyumba, T.O., Wilson, K., Derrick, C.J., and Mukherjee N. (2018) The use of focus group discussion methodology: Insights from two decades of application in conservation. *Qualitative Methods for Eliciting Judgements for Decision Making*. 9(1), pp. 20–32.

Pole, C. and Morrison M. (2003) *Ethnography for Education*. Berkshire: Open University Press.

Rudge, T. (1995) Response: Insider ethnography: Researching nursing from within. *Nursing Inquiry*. 2(1), p. 58

Shepherd, M. (2007) *Appraising and Using Social Research in the Human Services – An introduction for Social Work and Health Professionals.* London: Kinsley

Stanley, L. (2016) Using focus groups in political science and international relations. *Politics.* 36(3), pp. 236–249.

Stewart, D.W., Shamdasani, P.N., and Rook, D.W. (2007). *Applied Social Research Methods Series: Vol. 20. Focus Groups: Theory and Practice* (2nd ed.). Thousand Oaks, CA: Sage Publications, Inc. https://doi.org/10.4135/9781412991841

Wilkinson, S (1998) Focus group methodology: A review. *International Journal of Social Research Methodology.* 3(1), pp. 181–203.

10 Data Analysis and Trustworthiness in Qualitative Research

Christopher M. Hayre

10.1 INTRODUCTION

The process and application of analysing data and need to ensure research remains 'trustworthy' is by no means linear. As identified in chapters 8 and 9, we appreciate the flexible nature of qualitative research. For instance, it is generally accepted that different researchers examining similar phenomena may come up with different interpretations. What remains important, however, is that whilst the conduct and practice of research will vary, there is a need for methodological finesse, coupled with openness, honesty and integrity. By engaging in this way, prospective researchers applying qualitative research should feel comfortable with how data is being generated and later concluded. The primary purpose of this chapter, as well as this book, is to not only 'guide' researchers through the analysis of qualitative data but to ensure it remains trustworthy. Although trustworthiness is examined in the latter stages of this chapter (and book), readers are encouraged to engage in the analytical and trustworthy 'phases' in order to familiarize themselves with ideas, practices and behaviours. This will naturally enable critical engagement of behaviours, actions and reactions before, during and after any fieldwork. It is also important to acknowledge that whilst this chapter offers a single perspective via theoretical and practical experience, readers are encouraged to examine alternate (and seminal) texts in order to appreciate diversity amongst scholars historically and transnationally.

For data analysis, researchers share a common goal – uncovering original phenomena. Regardless of the approach, researchers intend to delve deep into observational or conversational data with participants in search for data that highlights unique and insightful empiricism. Further, appreciation of notetaking, sorting, coding, categorizing and thematic development remains key, with a clear emphasis on the role of the researcher. The term 'rigor' has been widely replaced with the term 'trustworthiness' in qualitative work, hence its use throughout this chapter. Subcomponents of 'trustworthiness' are then further broken down in a way that not only links to literature but also offers practicalities. For instance, ensuring that qualitative research maintains its credibility, transferability, dependability, confirmability and authenticity is not merely determined by theoretical propositions alone, it is the researcher that remains accountable with reference to his or her practices prior, during and beyond

DOI: 10.1201/9780367559311-10

the research environment. Again, the purpose and practice of 'trustworthiness' may differ amongst different researchers and those specifically focussing on radiography. Readers are encouraged, however, to examine the diversity and/or parity of forthcoming approaches in order to either support or build on from previous experience. Seminal works on the practice and application of ensuring trustworthiness will help reinforce the value and importance of such practices, from a methodological and empirical standpoint and importantly help shape the practice and standard for determining 'trustworthiness' in radiography.

10.2 QUALITATIVE DATA ANALYSIS

Let us begin with a simple question: what is qualitative data analysis? As a researcher who has performed both quantitative and qualitative research, we should perhaps 'park' our quantitative thinking and understanding when thinking 'analytically' in qualitative research. At this stage, if having collected qualitative data, you will be faced with a large volume of information, deemed 'raw data'. This data may include observational notes, shorthand representations, verbatim words of participants and/or reflexive journal entries. At first glance, this information will be vast and have little or no order/relevance. At this point, it is the role of the researcher to not simply 'look' at the raw data but to try and understand it. To say there is a 'micro-method' or strategy that seeks to offer a step-by-step way of analysing qualitative data is not generally ascribed, which is naturally reflected in its uniqueness to both the research context and researcher themselves (Anderson, 2010). On the other hand, we must consider generally recognized approaches for performing qualitative data analysis in order for it to remain meaningful, transferable and accountable to the research project and indeed researcher.

A central premise of undertaking any form of qualitative data analysis is that data remains grounded by the participants in which the study serves and represents a culture or individual(s) in which the study seeks to investigate (Denzin and Lincoln, 2003). This chapter intends to reflect on previous practices, which have naturally been guided and developed from previous texts. This suggests that the practice of data analysis, itself, has an intentional and developmental phase. That said, for the purposes of researchers studying at undergraduate or postgraduate level, this chapter appreciates thoughts, complexities and uniqueness surrounding data analysis. Some common analytical approaches are identified to the reader and linked to an according methodology, which is typically applied within previous works.

10.2.1 COMPUTER-AIDED VERSUS NON-COMPUTER-AIDED ANALYSIS

The use of computers or 'computing power' to analyse qualitative data is not uncommon, and for some methodologies, such as ethnography, it may be viewed as superior (Allen, 2017). To some degree, it is likely that computers will be used (in some form or another), either via transcription, storing, securing or 'backing up' data. This differs from using computers to assist with the analytical process. Since the 1980s, computers have been used for qualitative data, in particular, due to the often large datasets unfolding as part of the qualitative work. Because of this, coupled with enhanced processing power, computers can process by inputting, analysing and evaluating data easier, and quicker (Rodik and Primorac, 2015). In addition, an added benefit emerges whereby upon working with multiple researchers, across multiple sites or organizations, the use of computers can centralize qualitative work and subsequent analysis, whereby accessibility is made on secured platforms. Whilst computers continue to remain significant in our everyday lives by facilitating professional and personal endeavours, they do have limitations. A central limitation of all technological devices and computers is that they remain tools. Like any tool, if applied well, it can be used to our advantage. However, if understood poorly, it will lead to an under-appreciation of the device. Whilst in-house training programmes for qualitative software packages are often available, users are still required to become familiar with the software and should dedicate time to best understand its features. Silver and Lewins (2014) provide a comprehensive list of computing programmes that can be used in qualitative data analysis, such as Hyperresearch, NVivo and ATLAS.ti. Like many software packages, each offers unique interfaces. Holloway and Galvin (2017) remind us, however, that whilst computers can be useful, the use of technology does not replace the intellectual and inherent process of reflection amongst researchers. This is an important consideration and previously highlighted in chapter 9 whereby reflexivity and researcher positionality play a key role in the accumulation of empiricism in qualitative research. Further, because computers are tools, programed to perform events when instructed, they will not arguably interpret data in the same way a human would. For example, would a single word, comment or sentence that has previously been suppressed or overlooked in the overall narrative or language be easily discernible?

The process and efficiency by which computers aid our practices are profound. Whereby copying, cutting and pasting enables us to (re)create files and/or make duplicates to ensure no loss of data. Another advantage is that data are stored centrally, i.e., within a single program or application and not perhaps 'floating' in a number of different files or folders. In my view, the value of computing programs becomes essential for inter-disciplinary working, coincided with cloud-based working, whereby computers act as a tool to facilitate communal analysis and arguably engages wider empirical interest amongst multiple researchers. Notable disadvantages of using computers for data analysis is perhaps something more methodological and philosophical. For instance, it is worth remembering that when seeking the use of computers, it should not be justified in the same way as using quantitative data. Quantitative data utilizes computer programs to assess large amounts of numerical data and perform statistical analysis in order to ascertain generalization. In response, qualitative researchers should not be inclined to perform more interviews than required if computer-aided programmes are going to be used. Here, we should be mindful of the methodological and philosophical tents of undertaking qualitative research in the first place. In chapter 2, the examination of interpretivist or postmodernist epistemologies appreciates multiple realities when generating original empiricism. Nowhere do we ascribe philosophical underpinnings that require 'generalized realities' in order for evidence to be justified. In short, a potential danger may arise whereby the collecting, analysing and evaluation of 'more data' is performed in response to tasking computers to 'do' the analysis for us and inadvertently seeking breadth, rather than depth.

10.2.2   NOTE-TAKING: A DATA COLLECTION AND ANALYTICAL PROCESS

Note-taking is a central part of the data collection process. It is used as a primary tool when observing and can be 'put away' when deemed appropriate (Emerson, Fretz and Shaw, 1995). In addition, it is also used during interviews or focus groups (Wilkinson, 1998). Here, whilst audio recording/video recording may be your primary tool, written notetaking is also valuable. The nature of notetaking, itself, is part of the analytical process, whereby the actions, behaviours and attitudes of participants are capture (Burgess et al., 1990) or utilized post-observation, in situations where the recording of information is sensitive (Hayre and Hackett, 2020). By simply deciding if/when to take notes, naturally becomes part of the overarching analysis. Whilst transcription may be considered as 'gold standard' seeking to capture 'every word' of the participant, written notes, in my view, remain an accurate and trustworthy form (Bailey, 2008). Notetaking, during the observations of radiographers, resulted in a number of exploratory questions for latter interviews, and without these initial collections, it would have failed to support or lay the foundation for constructive open-ended questioning, later recorded verbatim. There is perhaps a potential danger that notetaking is merely observed as a practical process and perhaps thwart with unreliability. On the contrary, from experience, the practice and analysis of notetaking itself, during observation, can offer detailed accounts of a culture previously underexplored, which is later supported with complimentary methods (Hayre, 2016a). After all, the practice of observation offers an inductive lens, thus notetaking arguably acts as a practical tool as well as an analytical tool, which may require refinement or action planning depending on the line of enquiry.

10.2.3   'GETTING READY': THINGS TO CONSIDER

The process of 'getting ready' will be an important step for first-time researchers. Before any formal analysis, it is important to ensure that data is stored securely, according hard copies remained in locked file cabinets, coupled with digital copies on encrypted devices to ensure no data loss. It is advisable at this stage to think about gender-specific pseudonyms (if applicable), but also mindful that pseudonyms can be traced back to their original source for auditing purposes. The first stage of analysis is to read or listen to raw data being collected. If observing, this may involve reading and recollecting actions or behaviours of radiographers. It may also begin by listening to audio recordings taken from semi-structured interviews. From experience and upon reading observational comments, derived from notetaking, this provided first-hand insight into radiographic queries or issues faced by radiographers during their day-to-day practices. These were often grounded on the participant's actions, behaviours and practices and not simply based on preconceived ideas. Moreover, upon listening to audio recordings of participants, the researcher, if transcribed by self, can carefully listen and transcribe audible conversations. The term 'verbatim' seeks to collect the 'word for word' narrative of interviews or focus groups. Often presented in a transcript and involving the participant and/or researcher/mediator(s) it can capture laughter, gestures, jargon or slang pertinent to the context. The purpose of narration is to retain the linguistic value of conversation between researcher and participant, as this can often provide valued insight of a cultural group (Tessier, 2012). In addition, and depending on dexterity and typing speed, transcriptions can be laboured, taking several hours, for every 60 minutes of audible data. It may be necessary to seek professional services, which will not only capture the information correctly, and most likely performed quicker. In some of my own work, the services of transcription were highly useful, especially upon working on commissioned projects whereby deadlines remain paramount, whilst also maintaining the empirical value of any conversation(s). Importantly, transcription services should conform to data protection and confidentiality practices, as governed by ethical approval. It may be necessary for typists to sign confidentiality agreements acknowledging data sensitivities and appropriate destruction of copies upon completion of any services.

If the researcher is listening and transcribing the interview themselves, the analysis will immediately begin (Saks and Allsop, 2010). By listening and typing the researcher immerses themselves in the analytical processes as transcription occurs and evolves, and thus, at this point, important to keep a separate document that contains emerging issues, ideas or opportunities. This offers pre-analytical considerations when analysing transcripts collectively as the researcher progresses, enabling an overarching lens on the emerging conversations upon transcription, see Hammersley (2003) for further justification. In addition, if researchers seek the support of a typist, they are likely to miss changes to the participants pitch, tone or timed response to particular questions.

During the transcription process, it is advised that 'line numbers' are used within the text. This is helpful in order to trace raw data, which may be requested at the publication stage, coupled with date, time and file name (non-identifiable) of the audio file or transcript. This facilitates our ability (as researchers) to demonstrate an audit trail at a later date, if necessary. It is also recommended that inaudible information is identified as 'UNCLEAR', supported with other labels, such as 'pause', 'interruption', 'emphasis', 'laughter' and/or 'coughing' when appropriate. The detail provided during transcription will help depict the conversation in its 'raw form' to any prospective reader and will remain vital upon analysis in order to understand and critique the researcher's questions, coincided with participant's responses.

10.2.4   The Beginnings of Data Analysis

A central part of all qualitative analysis is organization. For most qualitative researchers, the involvement of journal entries, observational field notes (audio, handwritten or typed), coupled with interview transcripts, to name a few, will remain paramount. From experience, separating data by 'method' will make the data more manageable (and perhaps more meaningful). Looking back, observation notes, interview transcripts and journal entries were placed in separate folders. This helped for two reasons. First, it offered a quick reference, depending on the location or topic of interest – an observational event or interview comment. Second, it facilitated the ability to examine data in a sequential phase. Although some overlapped is always inherent, for me, observational data facilitated inductive reasoning throughout. This was later supported with semi-structured interviews. The rationale for immersing in the observational data prior to analysing interview data was naturally grounded on the former influencing the latter – hence sequential. At this point, our notes should contain the time and date, coupled with location(s) providing an opportunity to make geographical sense of the data, especially if conducting multi-sited research. Moreover, as observational themes begin to emerge, some will naturally seem more important than others. Whilst these ideas are good to capture, it becomes supported or refuted with ongoing analysis, reflection and/or one-to-one interviewing (Pole and Morrison, 2003). Typically, then, whilst data analysis may be seen as 'separate' to the data collection phase, as considered with experimental research, in qualitative research, data analysis takes place throughout.

The process of observing, interviewing or recording/capturing supporting documentation will enable the researcher to have thoughts and feelings about what is being observed or heard. The inherent process of researcher positionality and reflexivity positions the research and researcher in an iterative state, moving 'back and forth' between each dataset, thus identifying behaviours and responses to events seen and heard (Kassan et al., 2020). This iterative process reshapes and refocuses the data collection process and also offers an analytical perception made by the researcher. In short, the beginning and ongoing process of redesigning and rethinking outcomes, albeit methodological or empirical, requires some form of analytical thinking and mindfulness to forthcoming developments. In addition, the process and use of journal entries are not only helpful to reaffirm or rethink data collection processes but also used to support evidence. Upon writing up your own work, it is not uncommon to include personal commentaries concerning a particular examination, or interaction with participants, or feelings pertaining to the research process. Below is an excerpt from a field diary used in the first authors PhD thesis:

> *Working as a radiographer I would initially use the similar functions available to me 'masking' improper collimation, pay little attention to the SID and rarely used lead protection on numerous patients. Upon reflection and continuous observations I realized I had performed and maybe even contributed to suboptimal practices thus facilitating the 'way things were done around there'. On reflection this allowed me to become part of the culture, 'fit into the norm of everyday practices', yet on the other hand by realizing my faults I was obliged to remain within my ethical boundaries and later began to take note of my practices, trying to apply stricter collimation, carefully select exposure factors and apply carefully SID positioning.*

Here, we appreciated the interconnection between emerging data with ongoing reflections. Naturally, it helps contextualize the researcher's thoughts and feelings at the time of observing, say, inferior radiographic practices, whilst seeking the betterment of practice. The scenario above, which took place in the field, is the active beginnings of data analysis for qualitative researchers, which supports and enhances the trustworthiness of data, a topic discussed in 10.3. (Friedemann, Mayorga and Jimenez, 2011). From experience, the possibility of failing to engage in such practices, with reference to sensitive topics or conversations with participants meant that as researchers, we may not always 'put pen to paper'. There may, at times, be conflicting ethical and moral duties to our participants that preclude notetaking from taking place. Thus, the act of 'doing nothing' in the field also requires reflection, which should be integrated. Whilst the beginnings of data analysis do not specifically detail a distinct methodological approach to analysing qualitative work, it is important because it nevertheless remains critical for understanding and evaluating the beginnings, or 'starting point' of generating empiricism in radiography research.

10.2.5 THEMATIC ANALYSIS

Thematic analysis is perhaps one of the most common forms of qualitative analysis and often applied to a set of transcribed data, such as focus groups or interview transcripts. First described by Gerald Holton in the 1970s, it is now regarded as a distinct analytical method for social sciences (Braun and Clarke, 2013). Typically, there are six steps to performing thematic analysis, which are discussed. The first step is *familiarization,* and as acknowledged, the foremost task in order to know your data (Braun and Clarke, 2006). Once familiarization has occurred, *coding* can begin. In qualitative research, coding is a way of highlighting aspects of qualitative data that 'stands out' as either important or worthy of examination. Braun and Clarke (2013, p.207) assert that 'a code is a word or brief phrase that captures the essence of why you think a particular bit of data may be useful'. For instance, the code 'suboptimum X-ray use' could be applied to an interview transcript, acknowledging deliberate incremental use of ionizing radiation in the X-ray environment. This could be juxtaposed with participants commenting on the intention to optimize ionizing radiation by lowering mAs, for instance, resulting in another code: 'optimum X-ray use'. Codes provide a shorthand method of capturing important concepts, ideas or practices within transcripts, which may naturally result in a number of codes.

At this stage, we need to examine the manuscript carefully and highlight anything that stands out. Because of the likelihood of uncovering many different codes in a single transcript, it is advised to use colour pens or pencils to trace and link similar responses to individual codes. As the researcher progresses through each transcript, more codes will appear either supporting or refuting responses by different participants. Both are critical. Once data has been carefully read, with relevant codes assigned, the researcher will be left with a list of different codes, colour-coded to reflect the opinions, attitudes or beliefs of radiographers concerned with a particular topic. This allows us to move to the next step, *generating or searching for themes.* At this stage, a long list of codes will have emerged through a critical examination of data. Again, Braun and Clarke (2013) affirm that pattern-based analysis allows researchers to capture original features of the data that help answer the initial research questions. It is here, whereby codes are assigned to themes. In the general sense, qualitative researchers can assign several codes to a single theme. In my example of 'suboptimum X-ray use' and 'optimum X-ray use', clearly, these codes are directly linked to ionizing radiation. Here, it would be sensible to assign these specific codes into an overarching theme such as 'ionizing radiation within digital radiography'. It is important at this stage to recognize that there may be other themes that emerge which may be linked to the practice and safety of ionizing radiation, thus belonging to the same theme. For instance, the use of lead-rubber devices or light beam collimation could also be encapsulated with the abovementioned example.

Upon the formation of thematic development, the researcher will have uncovered an array of varying themes that make up representations, codes in this case, of data. It is, however, important to return to the data and identify inaccuracies or areas that have potentially been missed. This is commonly deemed as *reviewing themes* (Vaismoradi, Turunen and Bondas, 2013). Here, researchers must remain critical of resultant themes ensuring they represent the narratives offered and whether any initial assertions of 'the theme' are still warranted. The goal is to not only review the thematic process taking place but also be mindful of exaggerating themes. Themes need to be grounded by the data, thus reflecting on codes and thematic development is important to ensure it does not lead to misrepresentation of data (Braun and Clarke, 2013). In short, the process of *reviewing themes* is reflexive and seeks to demonstrate how themes depict the radiography environment. The researcher should remind themselves whether thematic analysis tells the story of the research? Upon re-examination of raw data resultant codes and themes allow the researcher to take a step back and ensure the analysis is not only firmly grounded in the data but also relevant for the write-up stage (Braun, Clarke and Terry, 2014).

Before weaving the resultant analysis into a dissertation or thesis, it is important to define and name themes that have emerged as part of the research. Whilst at this point, the generation of multiple themes remains grounded in the data, there is now a requirement to *name and define* each of these themes. This may seem a simple process but in reality, researchers are required to formulate themes that not only represent data but also portray them in a transferable manner (Creswell, 2009). The themes also need to be 'punchy' in order to engage prospective readers, the production of a good story. For instance, does the theme fit into the overall story of the radiographic research and does it resonate with the initial research questions? The generation of multiple themes may lead to empirical crossovers, which can perhaps be merged or removed due to duplication. Of course, there is the danger of seeking to redefine or 'finalize' thematic development in order to represent data in a novel and interesting fashion. However, as appreciated in the next chapter, the undertaking of thematic analysis and data collection, in general, requires researchers to not only come up with original ideas and themes pertinent to the discipline, it also requires them to know when analysis should stop. Here, researchers should consider seeking feedback from academic supervisors, or via oral presentations at conference proceedings and/or discussions with peers in order to gauge a sense of peer review. The process of discerning the naming processes in thematic analysis offers an additional level of scrutiny in the analytical process, which upon reflection should enable researchers to become familiar with his/her outcomes. If, however, at any point the researcher remains unsatisfied with this part of the process, it is important to continue refining before moving onto the last stage – writing up.

The beginning of any *write-up* phase requires some discipline. During the early stages of writing up and amalgamation of empirical data it is important that authors are continuously guided by the data. It is recommended that authors begin by keeping the narrative logical, concise and pertinent to the context and scope of the project. In addition, most qualitative outputs in the field of diagnostic radiography (and indeed my own) will contain direct excerpts from participants. This is important because not only are excerpts kept verbatim, they provide a direct understanding and point of view of the participant. Further, whilst journal entries and observational notes are still relevant, clearly, any supporting narrative captured verbatim also enhances the credibility of a study. Presenting the participants' narrative alone is a powerful feature in qualitative research, but it remains critical to also provide analytical debate. For instance, are there any supporting or contrasting views from other participants? If so, what do these mean in the context of the phenomena being discussed? Here, researchers should avoid simply replicating what participants have said and offer more depth, seeking out both meaning and application. This may mean theorizing, reflecting on implications and potential outcomes, supported with existing literature. Writing up qualitative research should be considered as an engaging, informative and stimulating process that seeks to portray unique insight into phenomena or culture previously unseen. Researchers should strive to find a balance between offering academic finesse, coupled with good storytelling in order for findings to resonate and become meaningful and importantly, impactful to the radiographic community.

10.2.6 CONSTANT COMPARATIVE METHOD

A constant comparative method is a form of analysis that has its roots in qualitative research, typically grounded theory (Glaser and Strauss, 1965). As identified in chapter 8, grounded theory has influenced many researchers both historically and contemporarily. It is important to recognize that the development of this analytical approach resides in its iterative nature, whereby the 'pure' form of constant comparative method fails to exist in light of amendments depending on the goals or purposes of individual researchers (Glaser, 1992). The process of performing this type of analysis shares similarities with thematic analysis whereby coding is first initiated, followed by categorising, as emerging theory is captured. A key difference, however, is this notion of 'constant comparison'. By definition, the process by which semi-structured interviews are executed, such as sampling, collecting data and the overarching analysis are simultaneously undertaken until data saturation is complete (Glaser, 1992). By continuing with our interview example, it is possible to discern steps in order for prospective radiography researchers to engage, but also apply strategically. To begin, coding will take place, whereby narratives are compared with one another to form categories (Boeije, 2002). But as interviews progress in time, more codes will develop, some perhaps more important than others, leading to the creation of more codes and perhaps categories (ibid). Here, the process of *memoing*, the writing of memos remains an important feature in this type of analysis, but you will also note that these are performed outside the constant comparative process (Denzin and Lincoln, 1994). Memoing, then, is recognized as transforming theory, a theory that is superficial into rich original data. It acts as a process of theorizing the write-up of ideas about emerging codes and their relationship with supplementary data. Similar to my own experiences, memoing helped conceptualize incidents, such as 'near misses' involving ionizing radiation or adapting to different radiographic environments, coincided with knowing when and how to collect observational data.

This is clearly a data collection tool, whereby the absence of memoing would have naturally prevented the development of the method itself (Hayre, 2016a). This example recognizes the constant comparative method via interconnections between data collection strategy and analytical development, combined.

For ethnographic research, coincided with inductive reasoning, this type of 'grounded theory analysis' remained inherent in both empirical and thesis formation (Hayre, 2016a). The 'back and forth' nature between data and research methods remained a common theme during observations of digital radiography examinations. In light of this self-reflective development of both tools and data, a key category is often central, which I termed 'values and beliefs' (Hayre, 2016a, p.107), grounded by my own auto/biographical lens. It was apparent that my own values and beliefs led to the exploration of this topic and research of interest, which required reflection. Further, it is important to recognize that the 'core category' failed to remain 'static' but evolved throughout the research project because of life events and historical circumstances. In short, for constant comparative analysis, the core category remained pivotal in the development and theorizing about data in the radiography environment because it, itself, required a level of self-engagement to enhance theoretical development of empiricism.

In relation to coding, the process is similar to those identified in thematic analysis, whereby codes can be seen as identifiers to sections or segments of data (Strauss and Corbin, 1998). Importantly, coding for theoretical development may stem from a single word, phrase or sentence from radiographers. It may be assumed that 'more is better'. On the contrary, a single word or sentence can provide unique insight into a certain phenomenon, which may be supported or contrasted with other 'accepted' commentaries. Similarly, as identified in thematic analysis, the constant comparative method seeks to encapsulate common codes within a category, with the attention it remains linked to the core category (Boeije, 2002). Eventually, upon directly linking self (the core category), with the development of codes and categories, theory starts to emerge. Next, the process of theoretical sampling takes place whereby ideas are enhanced based on emerging data. This allows the researcher to think about his or her next set of questions or (re)visit a department to see how data compares with participants at other sites, notably multi-sited research. Here, the researcher is on an exploratory journey driven by the insights of others, which ceases when little or no further data is discovered, commonly known as theoretical saturation – the point in which nothing can be derived in response to the research questions (Glaser and Strauss, 1967). Ceasing data collection, however, may not be easy, which is discussed more in chapter 11. What remained central in the first author's ethnographic research was a 'grounded theory approach' to data analysis (Hayre, 2016a, p.59). Here, the purpose of the analytical process enabled the researcher to ask: 'do I have enough?', but also ask: 'is it time to leave?'.

The application and use of the constant comparative method has been widely applied in numerous contexts. Clearly, its use not only supports theory development but facilitates the development of methods. It was important in the work by the first author to adopt a 'grounded theory approach' in order to critically reflect on the methods applied in this underexplored area of diagnostic radiography. For prospective researchers looking to apply innovative qualitative approaches in medical imaging, coupled with a level of uncertainty, it would be useful to consider the need for constant comparative methods in order to interweave method development with the generation of empirical data.

10.2.7 ANALYSIS IN PHENOMENOLOGICAL RESEARCH

The process of analysing phenomenological research can vary depending on the 'type' of phenomenology applied. Few examples methodically exist detailing thematic approaches in phenomenological research in healthcare or radiography (Sundler et al., 2019). Central in this analytical phase is understanding the philosophy to which it belongs. There is, then, emphasis on prospective researchers not to simply understanding the ontological and epistemological principles of their participants but also apply these virtues methodologically to impart and influence the analytical process itself. In chapter 2, ontology and epistemology are detailed thus recommended reading prior to applying analytical approaches aligned to phenomenological data (Dowling and Cooney, 2012). For hermeneutic phenomenological studies, the traditions and practices aligned to 'thematizing' are recognized, helping us understand and interpret data by illuminating unspoken meanings of lived experiences (Sundler et al., 2019). The term 'Gestalt' is an analytical term and form of reasoning that focuses upon an individual's experience in a current situation and any self-regulating judgement(s) made as a result of the overall situation (Boris, Melo and Moreira, 2017). The Gestalt is an idea that seeks to embrace and gain a deep-rooted sense of the whole (ibid). In addition, the importance of 'bracketing' our own assumptions about a particular phenomenon is widely recognized in order to 'describe' and also 'translate' areas into insightful themes (Merleau-Ponty, 2002). This is further supported by Sundler et al. (2019) appreciating that researchers should strive to distance themselves from their assumed experiences of participants in order to study phenomena in a new light, making experiences 'more visible'. This is perhaps distinct from conventional thematic analysis or the constant comparative approach, whereby researchers are often 'closer' to the topic under investigation, coupled with preconceived experiences and assumptions of either the participants and/or the radiographic environment itself (Hayre, 2016b; Benfield, Hewis and Hayre, 2021). It is perhaps argued that our 'assumed experiences' of a radiographic culture leads to direct questioning about a particular topic – the placement [or not] of lead protection on patients, for example. Here, we appreciate the need for researchers to question their pre-understandings of the phenomena and made aware of how their ideas influence the analysis of phenomenological work (Sundler et al., 2019). The use of 'bracketing' can distance or separate inherent assumptions, although it has been critiqued. Gadamer (2004) argues that it is our assumptions themselves that remain pivotal to our understanding of phenomena, thus preconceived ideas will remain part of our understanding(s). It is generally accepted, however, that researchers become aware of inherent and pre-conceived ideas pertaining to certain topics, enabling researchers to set aside previously held assumptions about certain phenomena (Dahlberge, Dahlberge and Nystrom, 2008). In short, whilst phenomenological analysis remains inductive, a bottom-up strategy derived from the data, prospective researchers applying phenomenological methods may need to consider abovementioned analytical strategies, which encompasses both philosophy and openness with one's relationship to the phenomena under investigation. The work of van Manen provides a helpful examination in the work of phenomenological analysis, most notably interpretative phenomenological analysis (van Manen, 2017). In this critique, the work of Smith, Flowers and Larkin (2009) is identified, portraying this analytical model as an approach seeking to make sense of major life experiences. van Manen (2017) identifies the importance of turning to a phenomenon of interest with an inherent commitment from the researcher to understand that world fully. In general, we see phenomenology investigating the 'lived' experiences, rather than an emerging concept. In light of the 'lived experience', it requires the researcher to reflect on identifiable themes that detail the phenomenon, but one that is continually crafted and recrafted during the writing process. Importantly, researchers adopting this type of analysis, whilst ensuring they maintain a strong and oriented relationship with the phenomenon under examination, need to offer balanced arguments by recognizing significant empiricism and also 'the whole'.

Lastly, there has been some critique of phenomenological analysis, in particular, interpretative phenomenological analysis (IPA). It is not within the scope of this 'guided book' to delve deep into this debate, but important to highlight potential emergence and appropriate signposting for future researchers thinking about engaging in phenomenological research, and one that van Manen's editorial asks: 'But is it phenomenology?'

10.3 TRUSTWORTHINESS OF DATA

The rationale and practice of ensuring that qualitative research remains trustworthy will now be discussed. As we have come to appreciate within qualitative research, there is no one size fits all approach. It is, however, recognized that rigor can be maintained in order to ensure research quality is sustained. The term rigor is commonly referenced when identifying or labelling the need for quality in our research, however, in light of it meaning stiffness or rigidity pertaining to the methodological approach, we now recognize the term 'trustworthiness'. As identified in the previous chapter, whilst qualitative methods are commonplace, it does not mean it is practiced in the same way by researchers in different contexts. For most, we have come to appreciate this interchangeable nature and use, with recognition that trustworthiness is best prescribed to the qualitative setting. Hereafter, then, the term trustworthiness is used and accompanied with its generally accepted sub-features; credibility, transferability, dependability, confirmability and authenticity.

Typically, when thinking about trustworthiness it should demonstrate not just how the researcher got from one stage to another but recognize hurdles and detours along the way. A consideration for any new qualitative researcher is the peer review process for publication, which itself demonstrates variance in terms of 'how much' trustworthiness is included. For instance, reflecting on my own outputs undergoing the peer review process, qualitative papers have either limited (Hayre, Blackman and Eyden, 2016) or in-depth discussion concerning trustworthiness (Hayre et al., 2019). This is not deliberate, but often a reflection of varying word counts set by journals, coupled with required revisions from editors and reviewers as to whether more or less information should be included. The above papers, however, demonstrate little parity for new researchers perhaps reading qualitative articles in the same journal. It also leads to question: 'how much do I include about trustworthiness?'. For researchers reading this book, it remains a valid question and one that is perhaps unanswerable at present. What is needed, however, is greater reflection on qualitative papers passing the review process and how best to demonstrate parity in terms of demonstrating 'trustworthiness'. This also enhances the rationale for this book because not only does it seek to open up a much wider debate about trustworthiness of qualitative research in radiography, it also questions how it can be measured via dissemination. This may require discussion amongst editorial board members, but for now, and for the purposes of this book, detailed accounts are discussed for students, which may be useful in prospective dissertation or thesis writing and provide insight as to how prospective researchers approach trustworthiness.

To begin, we should acknowledge the seminal work of Lincoln and Guba (1985, p.290), whom sought to explain the fundamental purpose of trustworthiness:

How can an inquirer persuade his or her audiences (including self) that the findings or an inquiry are worth paying attention to, worth taking account of?

This statement illustrates a fundamental premise for qualitative researchers; how would your study be considered amongst your peers and whether, under scrutiny, does it add value to the discipline? This may seem like a harsh and perhaps pessimistic view that qualitative research needs to 'hold up' in the radiography community, but growing utilization and application of qualitative work does not always mean acceptance. This does not seek to dismiss or devalue the nature of qualitative research, say, over quantitative work, but provide a foundation – one that seeks openness, honesty and integrity in the practice of qualitative research in radiography. Five key areas, which can help ensure our project(s) remain trustworthy will now be discussed and reflected upon, from participation and commitment to the topic.

10.3.1 CREDIBILITY

The term 'credible' is defined as the ability to believe or convince a reader that the empirical work uncovered has actually taken place (Kreftin, 1991). One of the most critical aspects of determining credibility, then, is the practice of member checking. This is widely recognized by authors transnationally and also advocated by Lincoln and Guba (1985), whereby researchers seek confirmation from their participants in order to verify findings and ensure it represents their intended meaning. Member checking is generally achieved upon seeking confirmation of interviewee responses or multiple responses in a focus group or interview setting (Sharts-Hopko, 2002). This can often be confirmed by allowing participants to review verbatim words from transcripts and allow them to question or highlight discrepancies with what has been said. From experience, it is recommended that researchers either seek appropriate transcription services or provide timely transcriptions after conducting interviews or focus groups. This is important because if considerable time has passed, participants may be unable to recall responses and/or discussions between themselves and the researcher. Thus, in order to maintain good credibility, it is advised that transcriptions and member checking are performed in a timely manner, allowing the member checking process, itself, to become reliable.

Another area of member checking indirectly linked to interview techniques is associated with participant observation. For instance, in my own research, the use of participation observation informed the interview schedule. For example, it was impractical to 'member check' handwritten and often 'scribbled' notes collected during participant observations; however, the interview schedule arguably reflects the credibility of observations. One stark example is reflected in the style and type of questions posed to participants, directly linking observations, such as 'During my observations, I noticed the intermittent use of lead-rubber on patients, can you tell me why this may be?' (Hayre, 2016a, p.328). This question does two things. First, it focuses on an important observation made in practice. For instance, if the participant accepts the intermittent use of lead-rubber clinically, then it arguably enhances the credibility of the observation method and social construct made by the researcher. Second, the sequential approach of undertaking interviews after observation offered this open-ended question seeking insight into the phenomena itself. Thus whilst onus and significance of member checking may be performed post-interviewing, it can also be applied before and during sequential phases of the qualitative research via the engagement of reflexivity whereby analysis shapes the development of questioning.

The enhancement of credibility resides in time spent in the field. For most qualitative studies, researchers are required to undergo prolonged engagement with participants in order to gain thorough exposure to the phenomena (Denzin and Lincoln, 1994). Not only does prolonged engagement remain critical for enabling the researcher to become familiar with the environment and with his/her participants, but also critiques the researcher's presence in the field. Latter components whereby reflexivity and positionality remain central are also used to evaluate influences of the researcher whereby it leads to the generation of data (Hayre and Strudwick, 2019). Looking back on my role as a practicing radiographer, educator and researcher, this naturally required a multifaceted engagement, which was perhaps beyond the 'normal' realms of any sole research role. Whilst at times, the role became blurred, interviewing participants one day and then working alongside them on another (Hayre, 2016a), this did help build rapport in the field. The use of critical reflexivity, in this case, enabled acknowledgment of hypocrisy, enabling it to support the methodology and empirical data. The balance, then, between maintaining professional relationships, friendships, and researcher-participant encounters were all part of the research process (Hayre and Strudwick, 2019). Whilst conscious of 'going native', there were occasions where it became accepted, and on other occasions, avoided. The importance of enhancing and maintaining credibility may not simple derive from the data itself, but also via interactions within this multivariate role in which data collection takes place in particular, as boundaries between the researcher, colleagues and friends became whole.

Other forms of credibility can be found. For example, the natural process of post-empirical discussions with academic colleagues, supervisors, radiographers or fellow students enables the researcher to engage in a self-evaluative narrative with members of their academic, professional or personal community. This in turn allows the researcher to evaluate responses received, not just from participants but responses from his/her peers. These ongoing discussions and assessments not only support the development of an overarching discourse of emerging data, but also acts as a form of triangulation whereby a range of responses either support or critique forthcoming evidence. In short, the process and practice of credibility moves beyond member checking within radiography research via thought-provoking discussions amongst different members within the academic and radiography workforce. After all, it is often the radiographers themselves that identify unique and insightful data.

10.3.2 TRANSFERABILITY

When considering the importance of transferability in qualitative work, it is generally considered how it will resonate with our audience outside the research field (Lincoln and Guba, 1985). Because qualitative research typically involves small sample sizes with one or two locations, it is important that prospective readers resonate with the phenomena and context under examination. Methodologically, then, it is critical for researchers to describe the context in which the research is taking place. In radiography, this is closely linked to environmental and technological factors; it can also be linked to specific imaging examinations and/or patient preparations, which may also resonate with colleagues nationally or transnationally. The abovementioned 'thick description' allows a reader to assess and evaluate the contextual significance for their own practices (Becker et al., 1961). For instance, in my own research examining the use of digital equipment in general radiography, which accommodates a large portion of examinations undertaken worldwide is naturally proffered to have 'wide appeal'. Although the findings of qualitative studies have no intention of 'generalizing' nor be widely applicable to other contexts, this does not mean it fails to resonate with peers on a large, yet unmeasurable scale. In my view, whilst the undertaking of qualitative research sought to examine the experiences of radiographers in several hospital locations in the United Kingdom (Hayre, 2016a), it may still resonate with radiographers worldwide. Thus, whilst generalizations are not plausible by statistic inference alone, qualitative research plays a critical role in resonating with an audience that is not confined to the location itself. Further, as appreciated in the next chapter, the natural process and practice of reflection via continued professional development amongst healthcare practitioners, it is not unreasonable to accept an inherent self-examination and self-exploration as a result of reading qualitative research. This, in turn, postulates an unmeasurable form of generalizability and transferability via the process of learning, observing and actioning.

When ensuring transferable findings, it is important to provide as much contextual information about the participants as possible. Researchers will naturally seek a balance between ensuring anonymity, as outlined in chapter 4, whilst providing 'some description'. In my view, it will depend on the context and nature of the qualitative work and its locality. In general, however, it is important for researchers to provide description of, say, a radiographers rank, years of experience and/or place of education (domestic or international) in order for readers to critically 'place' the academic topic and responses of the participant, such as clinical competencies. The caveat, however, is the possibility of indirectly identifying participants or workplaces, either by geographical location and/or job description, as described earlier in this book. In short, the identification or participants and the workplace must be avoided, thus critical to provide descriptive transferable information that carefully considers the participants in order for data to have meaning. In all situations, researchers have a duty to their participants and organizations by ensuring identities are not fully disclosed, albeit directly or indirectly.

The practice of further enhancing 'qualitative transferability' can be found in the undertaking of multi-sited research (Marcus, 1998). As indicated in chapter 9, whilst the practice of multi-sited research offers advantages such as assessing and developing methods of data collection (and subsequent analysis), there may also be unforeseen episodes that lead to the cessation of data collection. Multi-sited approaches, then, seek to 'test' methodological strategies and alternate perspectives in different hospital sites. Looking back, the practice of multi-sited research not only provided greater depth to responses observed, it also facilitates juxtaposed discussions, such as sensitivities to the research strategy and proffered questions. This offers two learning points. First, the ability to capture varied radiographic workloads identifies that departments are culturally unique and its own 'way of doing things' in the practice of general radiography. This, in turn, reflects the ongoing need for qualitative research in radiography that recognizes the effect of workplace cultures and how these influence behaviours, attitudes and importantly patient care. Second, any opposed outcome leading to data cessation supports the notion that research may not always go to plan. Again, the multi-constructive experiences amongst participants and researcher highlight an unpredictable nature of human behaviour, which, on reflection, supports the value of qualitative research and examination of multiple realities whereby interactions (good or bad) highlight differences between individuals or groups performing the same task. In short, the differences captured aim to provide a more realistic perspective of varying imaging departments, which remain supportive to data generation by enhancing the transferability of a given topic.

10.3.3 DEPENDABILITY

When considering dependability as part of our overarching trustworthiness, it is important to think about the term. To be 'dependable' infers some form of reliability within the research design and its association with those 'methodologically practiced'. For instance, in order for qualitative research to be dependable, it should be driven by the research questions (Thomas and Magilvy, 2011). This may seem obvious, but as previously highlighted in chapter 8, qualitative approaches will differ depending on what is being uncovered. Importantly, ensuring ongoing reliability within qualitative work is having an acute awareness of reflexivity (Emden and Sandelowski, 1999). This is the most useful criterion when considering dependability, which considers the role of the researcher on the overarching dependability of a study. We have recognized the importance of qualitative work, whereby the actions, attitudes and behaviours influence the actions of others. Thus upon entering the research field and analytical process via inductive reasoning, it will remain iterative as the researcher continues to operate. Throughout, the dependability of the research and researcher is 'alive', coupled with the myriad of interactions and interpretations. it is here where the journey of ensuring reliability begins.

The process of observing and listening to gatekeepers, participants' reactions, applying alternate data collection strategies and adapting both physically and emotionally are facets reflecting the dependable nature of the research. Dependability moves beyond the research space, whereby analysis, supervisory meetings and 'writing up phase' remain critical by ensuring dependability of the work. This does not presume it takes place in a rigid or linear way, it merely accepts that dependability within a research project begins and ends with reflexive thought-processes and actions throughout. Here, not only do we observe both accountability and integrity of researchers but also maintain our responsibilities. Critical in the abovementioned is reflected in open and honest reflections about the research process. To dismiss the notion of reflexivity would fail to recognize the role and impact qualitative researchers have on their participants and the environment. Further, the notion of reflexive actions or reflexive behaviours is interweaved throughout this book not as tokenism but as a self-critical tool recognizing development that appreciates a 'back and forth' lens.

An additional feature of dependability in qualitative research ensures it offers a sound audit trail (Murphy and Yielder, 2010). Audit trails are used in order to 'trace' assertions or commentaries made by participants or researchers. Audits are often used in radiography when assessing image quality of radiographic images. Using this example from practice, we know that a key feature of auditing radiographs determines clinical competency and accountability of radiographers, whilst offering support, education or training to areas of practice that remain suboptimum. In a similar fashion, the sense of 'auditing' in qualitative research can be viewed as assessing a researcher's accountability and competency. Here, it is important that researchers consider their 'auditable practices' early in their work and pre-empt review meetings to ensure tracing actions and practices remain sound. Examples include following ethical processes and documenting unforeseen actions, observations and adaptations in the field. Other considerations may involve narratives or commentaries made in the final thesis or publication. For example, can the researcher's assertions in discussions and conclusions be held to 'account' and traceable back to the participant's responses or observations? Such practices should provide the reader with confidence that assertions are built on sound methodological and empirical foundations and not merely exemplified to enhance academic gain. An example in my own work is reflected in the 'physical position' and 'presence' of the researcher, which impacted relations with participants (Hayre, 2016a). At one hospital, I was asked to wear a doctor's white coat, a practice not commonly observed in the United Kingdom, clinically. This attire (when compared to other hospital sites) altered my positionality. For some patients, I was assumed to be a 'medical doctor', whereby patients would ask for a medical diagnosis based on their imaging examination. Further, this also impacted upon radiographers, allowing me to stand out as a researcher. Upon comparison with other research sites, it offered greater opportunity for written notes and detailed observations. Importantly, the 'white coat' was not part of the research process, nor predictable upon entering the research environment. This is one example of maintaining dependability throughout the research process whereby alternate or unusual situations lead to different interactions and subsequent engagements with participants. By recognizing this methodological change, it can enable readers to gauge accountability from the researcher in the field and thus provide audit trails in which the researcher and reader can visualize.

For any prospective researcher, it is important to be mindful and also critical of similar events. Unexpected changes or occurrences in the field influencing empirical outcomes should not only be recorded, but welcomed. At the time, they may feel misplaced, odd or even inappropriate, but via critical reflexivity and recording of actions, events allow researchers to engage with such unique methodological accounts. This will help improve the overarching trustworthiness, dependability and accountability of the study that has taken place and allow readers to resonate with findings uncovered.

10.3.4 CONFIRMABILITY

Confirmability is regarded as a process whereby data is presented in a manner that does not impose researcher bias. Whilst there will always be some form of researcher involvement, one of the most obvious and perhaps rigorous methods of ensuring a lack of bias is by presenting voices verbatim. Regardless of slang, jargon, tone or curses used, the narrated voice of a participant not only represents the views and attitudes but also depicts the culture within which the narrative belongs. Importantly, then, for prospective researchers, transcription is critical to accurately depict participants' opinions in the qualitative process. As observed within earlier commentary, our data analysis strategies will determine the 'type of story' told, but central to this resides in the linguistic cues held by participants and how these are presented to the reader. In addition to this, aspiring to confirmability not only reflects consensus of a particular theme but also those juxtaposed from participants. This, again, reasserts the researchers' positionality towards emerging narratives acknowledging that not all participants feel the same way about a particular topic (Goffman, 1981). Whilst researchers should not seek to infer bias towards interpreting data, it also ensures researchers do not simply present the 'majorities voice'. The nature of qualitative research in radiography is not to seek consensus but provide original perspectives, even those identified against convention. In my view, this perspective not only satisfies the argument of remaining unbiased by the researcher but also demonstrates an appreciation of varied responses and values individuals hold.

Looking back on experience, which is evident throughout this book, any outcome of qualitative work resides in the perspective brought to a study. By accepting and engaging on 'who I was', and the role played during the study, I sought to distance myself from participants and topics. Here, readers should be able to determine 'methodological surprises', deemed 'methodologically relevant' to the research setting. Any shortcomings, potential misjudgements and/or areas of strengths should be overt and understood by readers, as it remains a central component of the methodological processes.

10.3.5 AUTHENTICITY

Authenticity is now a common feature when ascertaining trustworthiness. Whilst a 'late edition' by Guba and Lincoln (1989), there are a number of contemporary examples that help understand 'authenticity', which readers are directed (see. Shannon and Hambacher, 2014; Amin et al., 2020). The concept of authenticity, or to 'authenticate', can be described as showing (something) to be genuine or valid. Whilst likely to be protracted over time, it has relevance for prospective researchers in being able to strengthen prospective and current studies by either thinking or engaging in practices that 'authenticate' outcomes. For instance, pursuing authenticity amongst researchers arguably seeks to validate research outcomes not only confirming originality but also sincerity (Guba and Lincoln, 1989). This is important because it may reflect the lived experiences of participants with respect to the social-cultural practices of radiographers transnationally. Here, whilst authenticity is considered part of methodological rigor, it is focused on 'value', i.e., impact and how it benefits stakeholders.

There are five sub-divisions within authenticity that are important to recognize. First, 'fairness' requires qualitative researchers to ensure participants have equal access to the research and method of inquiry (Guba, 2004). This is important to discuss. For instance, researchers can often be poised between publishing in high ranking journals with associated high impact and high quartile status. This may bring benefits to the researcher/author(s), especially in organizations that seek publication in Q1 journals (top 25%) for promotional gain. There is also a caveat. Less ranked journals, with lower impact factors and quartile status, whilst may not be 'academically pleasing' for promotional committees, they may have greater significance in terms of authentic outcomes. At the time of writing this book, professional journals in radiography are often regarded as 'low impact' and 'low ranked', but professionally and academically affiliated to professional bodies to which practicing radiographers subscribe. This arguably offers greater 'fairness' for members of the community in which the research took place for members subscribing to the professional body (and journal) thus making the research 'more accessible' to members of that community.

The second and third are linked to educational and ontological perspectives. The former seeks to offer some informative evidence that can influence teaching and learning. Whilst this may be evident in self-educational practices, it is also important that findings have educational transferability beyond the realms of the researcher's own educational practices (Amin et al., 2020). The latter considers ontological viewpoints of readers and as identified in chapter 2, examines our existence on observed phenomena and thus important to help participants develop a greater understanding of the social context being studied (Lincoln and Guba, 1985). The ontological recognition of a study should naturally raise awareness whereby readers reflect on the viewpoints of people other than their own. This is important in light of the need for more qualitative research in radiography (Bolderston, 2014), whereby the experiences of some can be learned and reflected upon by others. This, in turn, also offers a 'radiographic appreciation' of alternate cultures, workplace practices and opinions of radiographers that were perhaps previously unseen. Further, whilst considered to offer original perspectives to others, other than the researcher, it is important to note that onto-logical and educational shifts can occur amongst researchers (Amin et al., 2020). Thus, whilst the researcher has enhanced their body of knowledge coupled with self-development, there will naturally be greater appreciation for how others (participants and others) view and interpret the world around them.

The last two criteria are known as catalytic and tactical authenticity. The former resonates with how well the research has led or stimulated some form of practical application (Guba, 2004). One obvious example in radiography may be amendments or new radiographic protocols, influenced by policy decisions, which are considered heightened forms of catalytic authenticity in radiography, for instance. The latter, tactical authenticity, is concerned with disseminating evidence that can empower stakeholders or colleagues to act (Guba, 2004). This may involve outcomes of inductive qualitative research, which is later re-examined or developed to explore, say, quantitative outcomes. In short, the relevance of qualitative research not only seeks to generate further discussion but may lead to the development of other empiri-cism, informing education and practice. It also seeks to empower individuals. In chapter 8, 'action research' was introduced, which typically sought to invoke some form of change to those suppressed or underrepresented. Thus evidence allowing those ordinarily suppressed to emerge via methodological tactics also demonstrates tactical authenticity (Moravcsik, 2014). It is within this space that qualitative research not only changes but releases or uncovers unspoken behaviours, leading to change. The power of qualitative research, then, seeks to uncover and lead its audience to demonstrate and highlight change, which can be seen as superior or inferior. For either, its purpose is the betterment of the individuals in which the research seeks to serve, our patients.

10.4   CHAPTER SUMMARY

This chapter began by introducing qualitative data analysis whilst considering computer-aided and non-computer-aided software. As a user of each method, there are distinct advantages and disadvantages depending on the study's intention and collaborative involvement. This chapter acknowledges that data analysis takes place as soon as the researcher enters the field. Being aware of our methodological pos-ition, coincided with emerging challenges or alterations will remain integral to the research process and to the analysis. Here, we observe the beginnings of organizing, sorting and transcribing as well as linking three analytical processes – thematic analysis, constant comparative analysis and analysis aligned to phenomenological research. Further, although a general 'theme' can be gleamed from these approaches, the deep-rooted experiences of individuals remain paramount, coupled with intricate differences between the methods of analysis, which readers will find helpful.

The latter part of this chapter focused on introducing trustworthiness to the reader. As acknowledged, the five critical components appreciate how 'rigor' can be achieved in qualitative work. Some may be more aligned to affirming what the participants have said, whilst others are interested in how the researcher has recorded and perhaps imparted change in the field. Either way, each sub-section carries its own form of practice when critiquing the practice and application of qualitative research. The later addition, authenticity, seeks to document wider scholarly appreciation within the radiographic community in which the research serves. For instance, ontological reflections, educational impact and possible socio-cultural change are now common place and aspired.

For any new qualitative researcher, the abovementioned tools and strategies may remain alien. Yet, the overarching purpose of this chapter has not simply been to introduce such terms, with a radiographic lens, but also to engage them from a practical standpoint, whilst linking to seminal works with the overall intention to develop and build on the development of trustworthy practices in radiographic research.

KEY TERMS

Audit: an independent examination of research information of any stage of the research process.

Bias: is regarded as a disproportionate weight in favour of or against a thing or practice. Researchers may bias towards topics of interest or ways of interpreting data.

Constant comparative analysis: is a method of analysis that uses inductive reasoning in order to categorize and compare qualitative data. It is focused on analysing data coupled with qualitative instrumentation, which can be reshaped.

Data saturation: is the stage in any research process that is no longer identifying new information. At this point, it is important for the research to stop data collection as little or no new information is found.

Iterative: is a process that is repetitive in order to generate an outcome. The overall sequence will end, but there may be numerous iterations before the process is ceased.

Linguistic: relates to the scientific study of language and typically involves analysis of language formation, meaning and context. It can be attributed to social, cultural and historical features, which have or continue to influence the language itself.

Member checking: can also be known as informant feedback and is a technique employed by most qualitative researchers whereby transcripts are sent to participants to verify narrated conversations and discussions with researchers and their participants.

Memoing: is the practice of recording notes about qualitative research. They are often critical notes containing elements of interactions with participants and/or especially with the researcher and his/her emerging data.

Pseudonym: is an alias, a fictitious name given to a participant in order to conceal their identity. It will differ from the 'true name' in order to protect the participant, abiding by ethical codes of practice.

Raw data: is also known as primary data. It is data collected at 'the source' and for qualitative research involves data from participants. It may be presented in a number of ways and primarily the role of the researcher to organize and apply meaning to the data.

Reflexive journal: is a tool that qualitative researchers use to capture ongoing events throughout the research process. It can be later used during data analysis and in the thesis development.

Rigor: is commonly used in order to identify strictness or stiffness. It seeks to offer an approach in research that facilitates consistency using a predefined framework, which can be internally and externally examined where applicable.

Shorthand representations: have been found helpful in the first author's work whereby the collection of radiographic actions are often fast. Symbols were often created in order to depict and recollect the actions of radiographers at later stages of the analysis.

Thematic analysis: is perhaps the most common form of analysis in qualitative research. It seeks to identify and uncover patterns of behaviour amongst individuals or groups and provide depth to the qualitative data.

Theoretical saturation: is a term that is generally used in grounded theory data analysis meaning that researchers reach a point in their analysis whereby data no longer generates more information to the initial research questions.

Transcript: in research refers to a written version of originally presented material, such as an audio recording of an interview or a focus group. The transcript is used in data analysis and seeks to present the words of participants verbatim.

Triangulation; in research seeks to utilize several methods in order to support data generated by a sole method. This can involve, observations, interviews and documents; it can also include mixed-method approaches, such as observation, interviews and X-ray experiments.

EXERCISES AND STUDY QUESTIONS

1   Upon deciding to undertake qualitative research, think about the context of research, i.e., where and how the research will take place and with whom. You will need to think carefully about 'when' data analysis will begin and be mindful of how you recorded this.

2   In order to question the researcher's trustworthiness, it will be imperative to remain open and honest with the progression of research. In this regard, be mindful of ensuring that participants are given enough time to 'check' what may have been said. In addition, it will be important to find a balance between 'familiarity' and 'strangeness' when seeking to remain close but also distanced from interactions and situations.

3   The analytical and trustworthiness stages of qualitative research are naturally interweaved. Whilst they are documented separately, here, it is advised that prospective researchers become familiar with them independently. At this point, researchers will be able to appreciate and the capture opportunities or challenges that emerge along the way.

REFERENCES

Allen, M. (2017) *The Sage Encyclopedia of Communication Research Methods* (Vols. 1–4). Thousand Oaks, CA: Sage Publications, Inc.

Amin, M.E.K., Norgaard, L.S., Cavaco, A.M., Witry, M.J., JHillman, L., Cernasev, A., and Desselle, S.P. (2020) Establishing trustworthiness and authenticity in qualitative pharmacy research. *Research in Social and Administrative Pharmacy*, 16(10), pp. 1472–1482.

Anderson, C. (2010) Presenting and evaluating qualitative research. *American Journal of Pharmaceutical Education,* 74(8), pp. 141.

Bailey, J. (2008) First steps in qualitative data analysis: transcribing. *Family Practice,* 25 (2), pp. 127–131.

Becker, H. Geer, B,, Hughes, E.C., and Strauss, A.L. (1961) *Boys in White – Student Culture in Medical School.* New Brunswick: Transaction Publishers.

Benfield, S. Hewis, J., and Hayre, C.M. (2021) Investigating perceptions of 'dose creep' amongst student radiographers: A grounded theory study. *Radiography*, 27(2), pp. 605–610.

Boeije, H. (2002) A purposeful approach to the constant comparative method in the analysis of qualitative interviews. *Quality and Quantity.* 36(1), pp. 391–409.

Bolderston, A (2014) Five percent is not enough! Why we need more qualitative research in the medical radiation sciences. *Journal of Medical Imaging and Radiation Sciences*, 45(1), pp. 201–203.

Boris, G., Melo, A, and Moreira, V. (2017) Influence of phenomenology and existentialism on Getalt therapy. *Estudo de Psicolagio.* 34(4), pp. 476–486.

Braun, V., and Clarke, V. (2013). *Successful Qualitative Research: A Practical Guide for Beginners.* London, UK: Sage.

Braun, V. and Clarke, V. (2006) Using thematic analysis in psychology. *Qualitative Research in Psychology.* 3, pp. 77–101.

Braun, V., Clarke, V., and Terry, G. (2014). Thematic analysis. In P. Rohleder and A. Lyons (Eds.), *Qualitative Research in Clinical and Health Psychology.* Basingstoke, UK: Palgrave MacMillan.

Burgess, R.G. (1990) *Studies in Qualitative Methodology – Reflections on Field Experience.* London: JAI Press Inc.

Creswell, J. W. (2009). *Research Design: Qualitative, Quantitative and Mixed Method Approaches.* Thousand Oaks, CA: Sage.

Dahlberg, K., Dahlberg, H., and Nystrom, M. (2008) *Reflective Lifeworld Research.* Lund, Sweden: Studentlitteratur.

Denzin, N.K. and Lincoln, Y.S. (Eds.) (1994). *Handbook of Qualitative Research.* Thousand Oaks: Sage.

Denzin, N.K., and Lincoln, Y.S. (Eds.) (2003). *Introduction. The Discipline and Practice of Qualitative Research.* Thousand Oaks: SAGE Publications, pp. 1–45.

Dowling, M. and Cooney, A. (2012) Research approaches related to phenomenology: Negotiating a complex landscape. *Nurse Researcher.* 20(2), pp. 21–27.

Emden, C. and Sandelowski, M. (1999) The Good, Bad and the Relative, Part Two: Goodness and the Criterion Problem in Qualitative Research, *International Journal of Nursing Practice*, 5(1), pp. 2–7.

Emerson, R.M., Fretz, R.I., and Shaw L.L., (1995). *Writing Ethnographic Fieldnotes.* Chicago: University of Chicago Press.

Friedemann, M., Mayorga, C., and Jimenez, L.D. (2011) Data collectors' field journals as tools for research. *Journal of Research in Nursing,* 16(5), pp. 1–14.

Glaser, B. G. (1992). *Basics of Grounded Theory Analysis: Emergence vs Forcing.* Sociology Press.

Glaser, B. and Strauss, A. (1965) *Awareness of Dying.* Chicago: Aldine Pub.

Glaser, B. and Strauss, A. (1967) *The Discovery of Grounded Theory – Strategies for Qualitative Research.* New Brunswick: Aldine Pub.

Goffman, E. (1981) *Forms of Talk.* Philadelphia: University of Pennsylvania Press.

Guba, E. G., and Lincoln, Y. S. (1989) *Fourth Generation Evaluation.* Thousand Oaks, CA: Sage.

Hammersley, M. (2003) Conversation Analysis and Discourse Analysis: Methods or Paradigms? *Discourse & Society.* 14(6), pp. 751–781.

Hayre, C.M. (2016a) *Radiography observed: An ethnographic study exploring contemporary radiographic practice.* PhD Thesis. Canterbury Christ Church University. Faculty of Health and Wellbeing.

Hayre, C.M. Blackman, S. and Eyden, A. (2016b) Do general radiographic examinations resemble a person-centred environment? *Radiography*, 22(4), pp. e245–251.

Hayre, C.M., Blackman, S., Carlton, K., and Eyden, A. (2019) The Use of Cropping and Digital Side Markers (DSM) in Digital Radiography. *Journal of Medical Imaging and Radiation Sciences* 50(2), pp. 234–242.

Hayre, C.M. and Hackett, P.M.W. (2020) *Handbook of Ethnography in Healthcare Research.* New York: Routledge.

Hayre, C.M. and Strudwick, R.M. (2019) Ethnography for radiographers: A methodological insight for prospective researchers. *Journal of Medical Imaging and Radiation Sciences.* 50(3), pp.352–358.

Holloway, I., and Gavin, K. (2017) *Qualitative Research in Nursing and Healthcare.* 4th Edn. New Jersey: Wiley=Blackwell.

Kassan, A., Nutter, S., Green, A.R., Arthur, N., Russell-Mayhew, S. and Sesma-Vasquez, M. (2020) Capturing the shadow and light of researcher positionality: a picture-prompted poly-ethnography. *International Journal of Qualitative Methods.* 19(1), pp. 1–12.

Krefting, L. (1991) Rigor in qualitative research: The assessment of trustworthiness, *American Journal of Occupational Therapy*, 45(3), pp. 214–222.

Gadamer, H.G. (2004). *Truth and Method.* 2nd Edn. London: Sheed and Ward Stagbooks.

Guba, E.G., (2004) *Authenticity criteria.* In Lewis-Beck, M., Bryman, A., Futing, LT. (Eds) *The Sage Encyclopedia of Social Science Research Methods*, vol. 26, Thousand Oaks, CA: Sage Publications, pp. 404–406.

Lincoln, Y. and Guba, E. (1985) *Naturalistic Inquiry.* London: Sage.

Marcus, G.E. (1998) *Ethnography Through Thick and Thin.* New Jersey: Princeton University Press.

Merleau-Ponty, M. (2002/1945) *Phenomenology of Perception.* London, UK: Routledge Classics.

Moravcsik, A. (2014) Transparency: The revolution in qualitative research. *PS Political Science & Politics*, 47 (2014), pp. 48–53.

Murphy, F. J. and Yielder, J. (2010) Establishing rigour in qualitative radiography research. *Radiography*, 16 (1), pp. 62–67

Pole, C. and Morrison M. (2003) *Ethnography for Education.* Berkshire: Open University Press.

Rodik, P. and Primorac, J. (2015) To Use or Not to Use: Computer-Assisted Qualitative Data Analysis Software Usage among Early-Career Sociologists in Croatia. *FQS.* 16 (1). [Online] Available at: https://www.qualitativeresearch.net/index.php/fqs/article/view/2221/3758 (Accessed: 30/03/2021)

Saks, M. and Allsop, J. (2010) *Researching Health – Qualitative, Quantitative and Mixed Method*, Los Angeles: Sage.

Silver, C and Lewins, A (2014) *Using Software in Qualitative Research – A Step-by-Step Guide.* 2nd Edn. Sage Publications Ltd.

Shannon, P., & Hambacher, E. (2014). Authenticity in constructivist inquiry: Assessing an elusive construct. *The Qualitative Report*, 19(52), 1–13.

Sharts-Hopko, N.C. (2002). Assessing rigor in qualitative research. *Journal of the Association of Nurses in AIDS Care,* 13(4), pp. 84–86.

Smith, J.A., Flowers, P., and Larkin, M. (2009) *Interpretative Phenomenological Analysis: Theory, Method and Research.* Thousand Oaks, CA: Sage.

Strauss, A., and Corbin, J. (1998). *Basics of Qualitative Research. Techniques and Procedures for Developing Grounded Theory*. London: Sage.

Sundler, A.J., Lindberg, E., Nilsson, C., and Palmer, L. (2019) Qualitative thematic analysis based on descriptive phenomenology. *Nursing Open,* 6 (3), pp.733–739.

Tessier, S (2012) From Field Notes, to Transcripts, to Tape Recordings: Evolution of Combination. *International Journal of Qualitative Methods,* 11(4), pp. 446–460.

Thomas, E. and Magilvy, J. K. (2011) Qualitative rigor or research validity in qualitative research. *Pediatric Nursing*, 16(1), pp. 151–155.

Vaismoradi, M., Turunen, H., and Dondas, T. (2013) Content analysis and thematic analysis: Implications for conducting a qualitative descriptive study. *Nursing and Health Sciences,* 15(1), pp. 398–405.

Van Manen, M. (2017) But is it phenomenology. *Qualitative Health Research.* 27(6), pp. 775–779.

Wilkinson, S. (1998) Focus groups in health research – Exploring the meanings of health and illness. *Journal of Health Psychology,* 3(3), pp. 329–348.

11 What Next?

Christopher M. Hayre

11.1 INTRODUCTION

This chapter examines the 'what next?'. At this stage, I am not only looking back on previous experiences but also thinking what prospective researchers are anticipating during the process of finalizing their analysis of data, qualitative or quantitative. This chapter, then, is not simply about qualitative or quantitative approaches but offers an overarching perspective to research itself. This chapter begins by discussing the process of leaving the field. There is much discussion surrounding the importance of entering the research environment in the literature, with heightened emphasis on ethics, approaching gatekeepers and maintaining good relationships. However, little currently exists within the radiography literature reflecting leaving the environment. Next, this chapter progresses with a discussion around research impact, the conventions of how 'impact' is measured, and also, perhaps, unmeasured. The final two sections in this chapter offer some unique reflections of my own research journey; that of the 'reflexive practitioner', coupled with the monitoring process. Discussions concerning the 'reflexive practitioner' seek to enlighten prospective researchers via engagement of reflexivity outside the research field and highlight its application beyond research, within undergraduate curriculum. The latter warrants opportunity to welcome reflexivity amongst undergraduate radiography students, which conventionally utilizes reflection. For most, and indeed engagement for authors in this text, the process and appreciation of reflexivity had enabled greater learning and development through observation and self-examination.

11.2 LEAVING THE FIELD

The process of 'leaving the field' is rarely discussed in most radiography research and perhaps notably because onus and focus remains on gaining access. The 'act' of 'leaving the field' is, however, an important consideration and signposted in a number of examples outside the radiography literature (Taylor, 1991; Michailova et al., 2014). Clearly, the relevance and nature of your research (whether qualitative or quantitative) will depend on the level of engagement required with certain stakeholders, gatekeepers and participants. For instance, if performing experiments in a university

DOI: 10.1201/9780367559311-11

laboratory, the level of consideration for leaving the X-ray room, whilst important, is not comparable to engaging with participants in a hospital, coincided with Researcher and Development Directors, as experienced. As data collection comes to an end, there is often a feeling of relief in terms of fulfilling research obligations, whilst answering research questions (Hayre, 2016). The temptation for a 'quick exit' to begin engaging in the analytical process and decipher original outcomes may be welcomed, yet, at this point, it is recommended we also consider an appropriate 'exit strategy' before leaving the field.

Looking back, the initial feeling of sadness was evident. The research experience required close engagement with new acquaintances and known radiographic colleagues, some of whom I had socialized with during my time as both radiographer and researcher. These friendships and reunion of colleagues, with some, would cease upon reaching data saturation in both qualitative and quantitative parts of my PhD work. It was anticipated that upon leaving the field, it was unlikely I would either work or 'research' with these individuals with my intention to move into the academic environment. Although we may think the 'research process' should maintain rigor, whilst be succinct and timely, upholding professionalism throughout, there were also elements of fun. The use of humour and comradery was not uncommon in the everyday context, supported with helpful and progressive interactions. This may all seem arbitrary on initial examination, but, the role of the researcher, with his or her participants is naturally supported with memories and inter-personal relations. This means that our interactions and encounters with staff, participants, patients, and gatekeepers not only facilitates the success of a given project but allows us to 'join' participants in their everyday world. Thus, upon leaving the field, there may be an emotional disconnect with individuals (Kenyatta, 2017), which are methodological and empirically important. Through experience and upon leaving the field, it is important researchers thank staff, gatekeepers and participants in order find some closure, in order to ensure a smooth exist with key members.

Whilst the abovementioned reflections will be grounded by the researcher, it is also important that gatekeepers are appropriately notified upon leaving the field. There may be expectations held by gatekeepers before you decide to leave, i.e., some formal 'form filling' or conclusive meeting. For researchers involved in the exploration of sensitive topics with perhaps vulnerable participants, the researcher is more than simply a data collection tool. They may have offered comfort, support or advice to participants along the way and perhaps recognized as a 'friend' or companion. These experiences felt by us and potentially by others are important to reflect upon in attempts of maintaining a level of personal and professional politeness when exiting the field. In my own work, the use of social media offered a useful platform for maintaining contact with participants. Connecting via social media offered prolonged digital engagement whereby it became possible to engage with participants over longer periods of time. Social media not only offered 'distance' through non-physical means but also allowed a virtual sense of togetherness, regardless of career development or geographical location. Here, the use of everyday technology, coincided with mutual agreements to 'keep in touch' supported the rationale for connecting with participants in this way. A caveat, perhaps, is that whilst practical research and social components cease from a methodological and empirical standpoint, there is an argument that researchers remain 'active' by means of this engagement. Further, it is accepted that this may not always be practical, sensible or safe, depending on the nature and context of the research; however, 'socially' it can offer benefits beyond research-participant conventions via prolonged digital comradery whilst extending field relations with participants in radiography research.

This is, however, not to say that all research encounters are similar and that all exit strategies are identical. For instance, being asked to leave a radiography department (as identified in section 9.4) was clearly at the request of the gatekeeper [senior radiographer] on duty at the time. This experience naturally led to the immediate cessation of data collection, which upon comparison with other research sites remained opposed. This meant that rapport building, trust and/or even friendships within this space did not always take place. Other considerations may involve financial commitments to participants, if/when engaging participants via monetary means (Jones, 2014). Further, there may be agreements to deliver presentations or some form of continuous professional development as part of the emerging data. Such events may also be used as modes of member checking, enhancing rigor. Importantly, agreements and engagements with participants offer more than simply engaging with the radiographic community upon exiting the field, it enables a researcher to make ongoing connections with his/her professional community, which may not only lead to additional research opportunities but also sustain and build relationships between the researcher and their stakeholders.

11.3 IMPACT OF RESEARCH

Embarking into the research space for the first time is often incentivized by advancing the profession. It may be a topic that resonates personally or one that has been observed as we 'move' or 'develop' as a student or practitioner (as in the case for the first author). Whilst personal motives may exist, we should also consider our 'impact'. Research impact is widely recognized within academia and for 'budding academics', as we look to impart or devise change within our respective fields. Here, the term 'impact' is identified because whilst we may observe the impact, grounded by metrics, a counter-argument affirms that studies can still influence change by non-metricized means. Here, an interpretation of impact and how it may look for prospective students seeking to embark on their own research journey is offered.

What is now identified as progressive ambition is perhaps what many prospective students (even myself at the beginning of my own PhD) seek to infer by seeking 'real change' in our practice. Whilst this may be difficult, it is important this driving force instils motivation but reminded of pragmatics. First, 'quantitative metrics' remain high on most higher education institutions agendas, and whilst countries differ transnationally, a shared goal resides with 'actual impact' being outside of the academic context, i.e., in the everyday life and practice of hospital care, treatment and management of radiographic practices (Research England, 2021). For example, in the United Kingdom, the assessment of research in higher education institutions is commonly known as the Research Excellence Framework (REF) and is performed every 6–7 years (REF, 2021). For higher education institutions, this exercise presents case studies that reflect the themes of research undertaken within an institution (ibid). Upon submission, case studies are reviewed by panel members who assess quality, impact and excellence, which is ranked by star ratings 1–4*. This is an important metric in higher education institutions and one that researchers and academics remain mindful of. That said, whilst not overtly essential for new researchers to be thinking about REF submissions, it is important to identify current practices, purpose and exercises in which research is assessed in order to ascertain what value and impact meant in research.

For radiography, in order to consider what kind of impact your research may have, it is important to ask a pertinent question: who does your research benefit? Depending on your response, it may reflect the dissemination methods/outlets in which to reach your audience. Moreover, by understanding your topic and respective audiences it will likely depend on the type of outlet, such as a medical imaging journal. Although the 'impact', usually a measure quartile status, as identified previously may be low, it should not detract away from the journal's quality, significance or indeed role for the profession and/or wider academic community. Two examples whereby its role in the wider community are now discussed. In 2018, my involvement in an experimental paper examined the detectability of wooden foreign bodies using ultrasound as part of an honours project in the United Kingdom (Mercado and Hayre, 2018). The study's intention was to challenge the referral pathway in medical imaging by assisting with the detectability of wooden splinters using ultrasound, instead of X-rays. Whilst a topic relevant to radiography, and subsequently published, it has also been cited outside of the radiography profession, notably those specializing in emergency medicine and medical interventional work. Second, a more recent experimental study (2020) explored the impact of secondary scattered ionizing radiation following the placement of lead-rubber in radiography (Hayre, Jeffery and Bungay, 2020). Again, whilst its application remained focused on clinical radiography, it has been cited outside of our profession by experimentalists, namely looking examining the dosimetry and attenuation effects of lead-rubber. Here, we observe the cross-disciplinary utility of our work and value, whereby it facilitates the work of other scientists or health professions worldwide. Notably, then, as research in radiography grows, it will importantly remain impactful to peers outside our immediate field. Further, whilst studies are intended to expand our own radiographic paradigm, the knowledge clearly translates into other disciplines. This wider appreciation and inter-discipline expertise is perhaps an area that embryonic researchers may not initially associate their proposed research to affect, but with these examples above, it identifies wider impact, which perhaps would not have been thought possible.

A clear feature of assessing 'impact' using citation count is commonplace and thus a helpful tool for assessing the impact of work; however, there are other forms of impact that are transferable into the clinical setting. Before this is discussed, it is important to recognize this as a form of 'widening impact', which can be used to strengthen both rigor and trustworthiness in quantitative and qualitative studies. The most obvious method of achieving impactful outcomes is via academic dissemination in reputable journals. This peer-review process not only affiliates with reputable publishers via a non-predatory approach but also remains a proper means of sharing original work and thought-provoking ideas. This is often supported with an affiliation to membered organizations enhancing its credibility and applicability. This, in turn, offers members of the radiographic community the ability to read and apply research in their everyday context, but how do we measure this? For instance, if a radiographer reads a published paper and reflects (or becomes reflexive – as identified in section 11.4.), deciding to incorporate such actions into their everyday practices this remains impactful. Thus, because the practice of reflection is inherent within a radiographer's everyday practice, this will have an unmeasurable impact on the practice of radiographers. Whilst the number of 'downloads' for any given article can provide some indication, there is still some difficulty in ascertaining its practical effectiveness in medical imaging departments. To some degree, then, it is difficult to measure the actual 'value' and 'application' a piece of research has on a profession, such as radiography, especially as healthcare professionals are required to reflect as part of their continuing professional development.

An obvious example of impact concerns the development of policy, which can lead to changes in departmental protocols. On a celebratory note, an output stemming from my PhD helped support the development of policy in the United Kingdom concerning the placement of lead-rubber. The 'Guidance on using shielding on patients for diagnostic radiology applications' is a joint publication made by the British Institute of Radiology, Institute of Physics and Engineering in Medicine, Public Health England, Society and College of Radiographers and Royal College of Radiologists (British Institute of Radiology, 2020). On the one hand, this demonstrates 'impact' because it has the potential to influence change in local departments transnationally, if protocols are developed or adapted based on this guidance. On the other hand, however, whilst policy draws on existing evidence to impart radiographic change, there is likely to be disagreement with assertions made in the policy. It has already been proffered that radiographers may not be applying previously published evidence in practice (Snaith, 2016), identifying an apparent disconnect with implementing empirical work. This leads us to question whether such policy amendments will differ because whilst policy seeks to infer change, either via local protocol development and/or wider understanding, alternate ideologies in radiographic practices may still remain via social constructivist ontologies, leading to alternate decision-making. This leads us not to question the place of policymaking in general, but identify that in order for policy to improve the behaviour of its members, it may be required to monitor attitudes, ideas, beliefs and, importantly, clinical practice.

Research facilitating policy development examined the attitudes and perceptions of radiographers applying lead (Pb) protection in general radiography (Hayre et al., 2017). Most notably, the assertions made stemmed from qualitative research using social constructivism, accepting multi-variant realities whereby the practice of protection devices will differ from one radiographer to another. This leads us to assume that protocol development itself is not fixed, but based on the ongoing interpretations and behaviours of individuals. In short, we know that policy has the potential to influence change and practice behaviour, coupled with collegiality from professional groups. This is rewarding. However, we should remain conscious that where research influences decision-making to help inform widespread change, it should not discard the fluid and flexible nature of qualitative research. Through acknowledging the philosophical practices of qualitative research, coupled with collegiality and critical discussion, are likely to enhance patient care and safety in radiography.

11.4   REFLEXIVE PRACTITIONER

The importance of reflexivity during qualitative research has already been identified in chapter 9 and although typically associated with qualitative researchers, here, I wish to move beyond the methodological realms of reflexivity, but consider it within education. The 'reflexive practitioner' is a concept that has been suggested elsewhere, but little emphasis resides in radiography. Pollner (1991, p.370), for instance, defines reflexivity as 'an 'unsettling,' i.e, an insecurity regarding the basic assumptions, discourse and practices in describing reality'. Our everyday sense of the term reflexivity has enabled us to critically examine our underlying assumptions of action and the impact these have on a widened perspective (Latour, 1988). If we consider this concept alone, it resonates with most healthcare practitioners via a self-critical and developmental process within which we continuously engage. Here, the postulation of a 'reflexive radiographer' moves beyond the 'reflective radiographer' coupled with integration in undergraduate education. Currently, the education of undergraduate radiographers typically requires students to reflect, which is not without its challenges (Baird, 2008). Reflection, in the general sense, is typically something performed either in isolation, i.e., on a particular event or scenario (a specific imaging examination, for instance). This type of reflection is helpful for students because it enables them to focus on specific events, such as experiencing something for the first time, how they would manage it and what actions would take place if encountered again? Whilst helpful, there is a limitation with this type of reflection whereby it arguably works in silo, focusing on either a new experience, one which can be learned and developed if encountered again. Further, Baird (2008) reports challenges within which radiography education needs to critically engage and perhaps offer new strategies. As acknowledged, reflexivity is more than simply reflecting on a specific event that happens at a single point in time. Instead, it seeks to engage individuals over a prolonged period of time, drawing on experiences and events that take place along the way, such as the development and emergence/refinement of this book, for instance. Reflexivity enables us to critically examine 'self' on a continuous scale and often enables researchers to self-observe his/her interactions with participants and examine others actions or behaviours and act or react accordingly. In short, reflexivity is not looking at a single event, but a spectrum of interactions and incidences occurring over time. For student radiographers or practitioners, the former may mean a three-year undergraduate degree, offering a deeper and longitudinal event of self-critique. For example, if reflection involves recollecting an X-ray procedure whereby exposures were deemed too high the student/radiographer may consider whether their source to image distance (SID) was correct, whether appropriate collimation had been applied or whether the kVp/mAs was too high. These technical features are important for any reflective process to take place, whereas, reflexivity, on the other hand, would not only assess the technical components affiliated with the imaging examination, but examine deep-rooted questions, base values, culture, radiographer–patient relationship and overall competency as to why the exposure may have been too high. This asks more critical questions about the behaviour of suboptimum techniques because for reflexivity it does not discern events as 'one offs' but encompasses existential and inherent factors for the development and sustainment of improper radiation dose practice.

Looking back on my role as a radiographer, we perhaps inadvertently become 'critically reflexive' without fully being aware of it. For example, as radiographers [and researchers] we are continuously observing, learning and adapting our behaviours depending on the needs of the department, relations with peers and supervisors, accompanied with continuous self-examination. One obvious example is evident in the work of a locum radiographer. For most, the locum radiographer is unique because it requires radiographers to be adaptable to different workplaces and 'fit in' at short notice. It requires adaptation to local cultures and 'ways of doing' where necessary. It is also accompanied by finding a balance between acting and behaving in a professional manner, coincided with maintaining a certain level of 'friendliness' and 'good behaviour'. The locum radiographer is not only required to perform radiographic examinations in a 'proper fashion' deemed appropriate by the culture, but also sustain a sense of managerial expectation, peer acceptance, coupled with an overarching requirement of learning 'new cultural norms'. For me, the locum radiographer is continuously defining and redefining him/herself in different environments over a period of time, vis-à-vis reflexivity. This, in short, is an example of 'radiographic reflexivity' whereby adaptation to workplace practices, whilst ensuring (s)he plays their part remains part of their everyday environment. Locum radiography requires adaption, which provides us with some appreciation of how reflexivity has practical implications seeking to satisfy the role, but also the views of others.

Through observation and interaction, locum radiographers may interact with a number of staff, over a number of years. This may help define and redefine how our practices in radiography differ. The events are not, then, captured via scenario-based reflections alone, but through learned behaviour and greater awareness of our positionality, discussions with peers and observing the actions of others. If locum radiographers resemble a reflexive practitioner, this leads us to question its transferability for radiographers and student radiographers. Experiences of adaption, geography, interactions and actions with locum radiographers naturally resonate with varying placement settings for undergraduate students. The similarities offer opportunities for educators to not only introduce reflexive elements in their undergraduate education but allow the practice of reflexivity to take place, which is anticipated to support students now and in future years.

A central feature enabling reflexive practice and education requires individuals to look beyond the technical facets of our practice. Relying on technical aptitude can be misleading, as we have already observed with 'dose creep' (Hayre, 2016). In essence, a deeper and more critical self-examination of our moral and ethical behaviour is needed in order to situate ourselves independently from practice phenomena whilst also critically assessing assumptions of radiographic phenomena. As identified in chapter 2, this may require a subtle, but critical 'postmodern shift', which looks to not only destabilize current ways of reflection but allow radiographers and student radiographers to engage more critically in their everyday practice behaviours. This, in turn, may lead to alternate ways of knowing, understanding, practicing, and ultimately provide opportunities for professional development. Reflexivity does not need to be affiliated with interpretivist epistemologies alone. It can span the philosophical spectrum in order to help instil thinking for practice application and development. An obvious challenge in recognizing the value of reflexivity in undergraduate education may reside in the overarching assumption it resides with qualitative research alone, accompanied with an according social constructionist lens. However, reflexivity can be incorporated in undergraduate education and beyond, but there needs to be appreciation within members of the community it seeks to serve. The opportunity, then, is that student radiographers become more reflexive in their curriculum and offer longitudinal appraisals of practice placement, either via actions and behaviours of radiographers and/or self, or via an on-going and deep-rooted examination of observations on placement. For example, students may need to focus on examples that may feel uncomfortable in order to examine how practices differ. This not only educates the student, but anticipates them to sustain reflexive behaviours as their career progresses. Further, the move allowing radiographers to become reflexive will not only require a cultural shift but also a philosophical shift in education. Radiography is not just a 'hard science', but deemed as a 'united science', thus critical to remind ourselves of our social-cultural responsibilities and how these will impact on students learning and practicing in the future.

11.5   MONITORING

The inclusion of 'monitoring' has been added here as an area of consideration for prospective researchers. The final stages of research are important as perhaps the feeling of completion is near, coupled with recognition of an up-and-coming viva voce or other assessment. Here, I wish to introduce 'monitoring' as a later stage of the research process. Forthcoming discussions are based on experience, which are anticipated to shed light and also pre-empt heightened awareness amongst researchers. In general, it is important to remain accessible with participants, which is perhaps easier in contemporary years. For example, upon leaving the field, it could be regarded as 'final contact'. However, in light of a number of social media platforms available, as identified above, it can also offer a sense of 'research monitoring'. For instance, until now I remain 'connected' with participants, via social media. This offers an opportunity for participants to ask questions concerning outputs, which they have contributed. This ability to connect and share empirical work via social media is helpful and perhaps on some level reengages the research with his or her participants. It may also act as a form of 'peer monitoring' whereby as outputs are published, they can read those in which they have been historically involved, especially as it may have been several years since data has been collected, and then published.

In addition to the above, it is important to monitor 'self'. The 'self-monitoring' theory sets to deal with an individual's ability to control himself/herself and for those inclined to 'self-monitor', which naturally leads to high levels of self-examination (Snyder and DeBono, 1985). Here, then, it is argued that recognition of self-monitoring amongst researchers is important because it can critically evaluate social clues and care about social expectations. During the final stages of any research and in particular postgraduate research, it can be a challenging time. It is important, then, for those who have an increased awareness of self-monitoring may behave more sensitively regarding the mental process, instruction from people, and/or identifying important events (ibid). Unknowingly, at the time of coming towards the end of my own PhD work, there were a range of 'ups and downs' that we inadvertently self-navigate, which one seeks to manage. By continuously monitoring 'self', we can capture our productive and non-productive moments during the final stages of PhD work and reflect on difficulties encountered. Regardless of your methodological approach, the researcher remains key to completing their research journey and it is important to remain mindful and conscious of our own health, wellbeing and mindfulness to ensure we capture and fulfil the research project, and not simply its demands.

11.6 CHAPTER SUMMARY

This chapter sought to raise awareness around existential processes pertinent to the research field. For the embryonic researcher in radiography, concepts surrounding the researcher's duty to leaving the field appropriately are acknowledged. Further, suggestions about finishing the research are offered with emphasis on examining impact. I sought to introduce the term 'reflexive practitioner' and how this could be readily transferable in both the clinical and educational space. A general theme noted is the development of the researcher, regardless of the paradigmatic approach used. Because the author does not stem, nor affiliate to either paradigmatic tradition, but engages in both philosophical forms of evidence, this in my view identifies that reflexivity can play a greater role in quantitative and qualitative research. Further, it is proffered that it cannot only develop practitioners via wider criticism of self, but becomes integrated at an undergraduate level. By critically engaging with our observations, values and actions, it is anticipated students will be able to engage with topical phenomena through critical exploration of their own learning in both academic and clinical practice settings.

KEY TERMS

Citation: a quotation form or reference to a book, paper or author. In scholarly work, this often recognizes the value of a paper in its respective community, but either stimulating debate or used as supporting evidence.

Cultural shift: is a term that seeks to move culturally. It often requires a change in beliefs, behaviours and outcomes leading to successful and influential change.

Digital comradery: is a term that recognizes the idea of both engaging and creating a real sense of community and friendship, but via digital means, such as social media.

Exit strategy: For any prospective researcher, whilst gaining access is often the priority, it is also important to consider your exit strategy. For instance, when thinking about leaving the field, who you contact, how, coupled with exit interviews or written notices required to relevant gatekeepers.

Final contact: Here, recognition of 'final contact' is concerned with the physical 'goodbye' with participants in a research site. Prior to connectedness established with social media, the 'final contact' would have most likely been the final connection with any participant.

Leaving the field: Leaving the field enables a researcher to feel a sense of accomplishment but also ensures that they have notified all stakeholders.

Locum radiographer: a role performed by a radiographer at different hospital locations. A role that requires flexibility and adjustment to change, depending on local workplace cultures, protocols and 'ways of doing'.

Manuscript: is recognized as a written document, either a book or journal paper, but has not been published.

Mini viva: I refer to my experiences of being part of an ethics review panel whereby I questioned the methodological practices. A helpful exercise that whilst cannot be attributed to a 'real viva', but can 'test' methodological rigor of the overarching study.

Monetary: relates to money or currency and may be important if/when recruiting participants with financial incentives.

Philosophical shift: is a concept that requires alternate forms of philosophical thinking in order to accept or consider alternate discourses.

Policymaking: is the process of formulating policies that deliberately set out principles to guide decision-making and achieve rationale outcomes. It is usually a statement of intent and/or required action that can be implemented as a procedure or protocol, such as the cessation of lead-rubber use.

Postmodern shift: is a term that requires thinking beyond the modern realms of radiography. For instance, it may require a significant destabilization of current practices or thought-provoking concepts in order to alter or change practice behaviour for improved patient outcomes.

Progressive ambition: a concept that seeks to 'change the world' through our own research. Whilst ambition is key to motivation, it is important to remain methodologically and empirically realistic.

Reflexive practitioner: is a concept that seeks to engage pre-registered practitioners at critically observing, learning and self-examining actions. It seeks not to 'reflect' on individualist scenarios, but engage in a much deeper sense of self-awareness and the practice of radiography.

Research impact: is concerned with impact in academic work outside the community and one that contributes to the economy, society, environment or culture.

Social constructionist: is based on the underlying principle that people will develop knowledge of the world in the social context and that much of what we perceive in reality depends on our shared assumptions.

Social media: is commonly regarded as an interactive Internet-based application whereby text, photos, videos and other data are either generated or shared via online interactive platforms.

Virtual social network: is a concept that moves the researcher beyond the physical space and presents them in a virtual social engagement with his/her participants, ex-participants or prospective participants.

Viva voce: is a spoken examination practiced for PhD viva examinations. It will involve examiners that pose questions to the student, which (s)he is required to justify and defend.

EXERCISES AND STUDY QUESTIONS

1   You may be reading this book at the beginning of your research journey. If your research involves close engagement with participants and gatekeepers, it is important to consider how you will 'leave the field'. Perhaps, think about the processes of informing participants or gatekeepers and how the research process has ceased and what approaches may be used to share this information.

2   I have argued here that reflexivity will remain pivotal in all realms of research. Engaging in reflexivity not only allows open and honest reflections but can enable recognition of outliers or management of unforeseen events. Think about how you can capture your research journal, albeit a journal and examine your development as a researcher, regardless of the methodological strategies employed.

3   In a world of social media, impact and wider debate, think about your involvement with social media and how you intend to engage with your audience. This may impact decision-making with participants, colleagues, gatekeepers and PhD supervisors. Social media has the potential to assess the impact and engage with the wider audience, it will have methodological and potential empirical considerations for prospective researchers.

REFERENCES

Baird, M.A. (2008) Towards the development of a reflective radiographer: Challenges and constraints. *Biomedical Imaging Interventional Journal.* 4(1), p. e9.

British Institute of Radiology (2020) Guidance on using shielding on patients for diagnostic radiology applications. A joint report of the British Institute of Radiology (BIR), Institute of Physics and Engineering in Medicine (IPEM), Public Health England (PHE), Royal College of Radiologists (RCR), Society and College of Radiographers (SCoR) and the Society for Radiological Protection (SRP). [Online] Accessible at: https://www.bir.org.uk/media/414334/final_patient_shielding_guidance.pdf

Hayre, C.M. (2016) Radiography observed: An ethnographic study exploring contemporary radiographic practice. PhD Thesis. Canterbury Christ Church University. Faculty of Health and Wellbeing.

Hayre, C.M. Blackman, S. Carlton, K. and Eyden, A. (2017) Attitudes and perceptions of radiographers applying lead (Pb) protection in general radiography. *Radiography.* 24(1), e13–e18.

Hayre, C.M. Jeffery, C., and Bungay, H. (2020) Do lead-rubber aprons always limit ionising radiation to radiosensitive organs? *Radiography.* 26(4), e264–e269

Jones, M. (2014). Getting out: Leaving the field and reporting research in organizations. In *Researching Organizations: The Practice of Organizational Fieldwork* (pp. 155–184). SAGE Publications Ltd, https://www.doi.org/10.4135/9781473919723

Kenyatta, J (2017) Leaving the field: (de-)Linked lives of the researcher and research assistant. *Royal Geographical Society.* 49 (4), pp.415–420.

Latour, B. (1988). The politics of explanation: An alternative. In S. Woolgar (Ed.), *Knowledge and Reflexivity: New Frontiers in the Sociology of Knowledge* (pp. 155–176). London: Sage.

Mercardo, L and Hayre, C.M. (2018) The detection of wooden foreign bodies: an experimental study comparing direct digital radiography (DDR) and ultrasonography. *Radiography.* 24 (3), pp. 340–344

Pollner, M. (1991). Left of ethnomethodology: The rise and decline of radical reflexivity. *American Sociological Review*, 56, 370–380.

REF2021 Research Excellence Framework. What is the REF? Available at: https://www.ref.ac.uk/about/what-is-the-ref/. (Accessed 28/03/2021).

Research England. REF impact. Available at: https://re.ukri.org/research/refimpact/. [Accessed: 28/03/2021.]

Snaith, B. (2016) Evidence based radiography: Is it happening or are we experiencing practice creep and practice drift? *Radiography.* 22 (1), pp.267–268.

Michailova, S., Piekkari, R., Plakoyiannaki, E., Ritvala, T., Mihailova, I., and Salmi, A. (2014) Breaking the silence about exiting fieldwork: A relational approach and its implications for theorizing. *Academy of Management Review.* 39(2), pp.138–161.

Snyder, M., and DeBono, K.G. (1985). Appeals to image and claim about quality: Understanding the psychology of advertising. *Journal of Personality and Social Psychology*, 49, pp. 586–597

Taylor, S. J. (1991). Leaving the field: research, relationships, and responsibilities. In W. B. Shaffir, and R. A. Stebbins (Eds.), *Experiencing Fieldwork: An Inside View of Qualitative Research* (Vol. 124, pp. 238–247). SAGE Publications, Inc., https://www.doi.org/10.4135/9781483325514.n20

12 Book Summary

Christopher M. Hayre and Xiaoming Zheng

Our passion for writing this book has stemmed from our experiences of teaching and practicing research methods for the advancement of radiographic knowledge. Our involvement in projects and subjects transnationally provides us with a lens that appreciates the value of qualitative and quantitative research. Our experiences are not professed in an authoritarian manner, but held by egalitarian views. For the first author, having educated student radiographers in the United Kingdom and overseas in the United Arab Emirates and Australia, I have often found refuge from other pertinent texts that are prescriptively generalized to non-radiographic audiences. Our desire for writing this book stems from years of not only teaching research methods but also applying research methods transnationally, coupled with leading and developing qualitative and quantitative outputs. We also appreciate affiliation with socio-cultural experiences and paradigmatic expansion. This not only reinforces our own educational practices, supported with empirical examples, but also heightens our credibility in the research process. It is our anticipation this book will offer students insight into the theory and practice of research in radiography and act as a guide to those undertaking undergraduate courses, honours projects and those in the postgraduate space. This book does not seek to replace texts, but offers a collaborative perspective as both a radiographer [CH] and medical physicist [XZ] in conducting and publishing research of our own.

This book has also been developed to reflect a 'methodological strategy' from the perspective of the authors. The nature of writing, content development and development of self is a reflection of the engagement with research overall, even at its inception. This is why strong emphasis relies on reflexivity from the outset, as appreciated throughout. There is also a clear overarching message in which this book seeks to portray. The research and practice of radiography do not merely stem from a single science. This book appreciates that radiography is part of a 'united science', and recognizes quantitative and qualitative methods as pivotal for the development of knowledge. By recognizing our research on a united front, we may begin to appreciate the value, philosophically, methodologically and thus epistemologically. For us, this allows us to accept methodological practicalities and diversities within this paradigmatic approach, which naturally leads to vast empiricism. That said, whilst

DOI: 10.1201/9780367559311-12

this may become increasingly recognized, it does not mean it will always be accepted. Whilst friction may exist, there is a growing trend of appreciating mixed methods, encompassing alternate methodological strategies previously unknown. This should be celebrated as it will continue to influence and enhance our evidence base now and in future years, improving patient outcomes.

Finally, for those prospective researchers looking to engage in the research space, it is now your opportunity to engage and also be critical of your own research and the views of others. Be guided by your motives for pursuing and enhancing the radiographic evidence and seek out critical ways of doing, as well as knowing.

Index

A5 notebook 130
AAPM 80
Academic rigor 37
Academically pleasing 163
Acceptance 3, 6, 17
Accountability 17, 161
Accumulative probability function 93
Action research 109, 119
ADNI 88
Aesthetically pleasing 22
Aim 8, 39, 45
ALARA 86
Alienation 6, 136
ANSTO 83
Anthropomorphic 47
Anticipate harm 51
ARPANSA 83
Artificial intelligence 98
Artificial neural network 98
Assent 55
ATLAS.ti 147
Attire 51, 147, 161
Attractiveness 10
Audio notes 7, 140
Audit trail 149
Australian synchrotron 83
Authenticity 145, 156, 163
Autonomy 47, 53
Awareness of Dying 117
Axiology 17, 30, 112

Back and forth 4, 35, 150
Backing up 146
Bayesian theorem 93
Beam hardening 69, 94
Beneficence 47, 50
Body of knowledge 5, 39, 164
Body size effect 66
Bracketing 155
Broad knowledge 37

Case control studies 70
Catalytic authenticity 164
Categorizing 153
Causal relationship 63, 69
Cause and effect 7, 75
Ceasing data collection 154
Certainty 71
Change management 109, 119
Children 46, 55, 60, 118

Christmas party 129
Citation count 174
Classical mechanics 94
Clinical investigation 72
Clinical trial 72
Cloud based working 147
Coding 151
Cohesion 53, 121, 134
Cohort studies 70, 73
Colonialism 137
Community based participatory 119
Comparative clinical trial 73
Complete observation 130
Computer aided analysis 147, 164
Comtean positivism 52
Conceptualizing 4, 33, 43
Confidentiality 49
Confirmability 162
Confounding effect 84
Consent 46, 48, 52, 54
Constant comparative method 117, 153
Contextualizing 33, 35, 43
Copyright permission 56
Correlation coefficient 68
Covert 8, 49, 53, 130, 141
Credibility 145, 153, 158, 175
Criminal activity 128
CRIS 67
Critical analysis 9, 66
Critical realism 21, 28, 29
Critical theory 38
Cropping 130
Crosssectional studies 72
CT 17, 22, 52, 67, 71
CT dose index 81
CT dose phantom 81
CT imaging 86
CT numbers 89
CTDIv 89
Cultural norm 177
Cultural shift 178
Culture 6, 9, 18, 22, 46, 49, 111, 114, 120, 122, 123

Data analysis 145, 146, 149
Data collection 129
Data Protection Act 49
Data sampling 84
Data saturation 132
Data sharing 87

Decision criteria 71
Decision threshold 71
Declaration of Helsinki 47
Deductive research 98
Degrees of freedom 99
Dementia 133
Dependability 145, 156, 160
Descriptive 160
Descriptive statistics 93
Detectability index 101
Deterministic response 71
Diagnostic image quality 72
Diaries 7
DICOM 87
Dictaphone 130
Digital comradery 173
Digital detector 51
Digital radiographs 2
Digital Radiography Champion 10
Dignity 52, 120
Dipyridamole stressor 68
Disclosure 48, 49
Discrete sample 93
Dissemination 112, 121, 138, 157
Dissertation 9, 27
Diversity 11, 18, 112, 145
Doctorate of philosophy 15, 57
Doctors coat 161
Dogmatic views 2, 10
Dose 10
Dose optimization 65, 98, 110, 119
Dose power 66
Dosimeter 66, 80

Edmund Husserl 115
Educational transferability 178
Electron density phantom 67
Emotion 117, 136, 161
Emotional virtue 6
Encrypted devices 148
Entrance skin dose 84
Epidemiology 70
Epistemological theory. See epistemology
Epistemologically irrelevant 136
Epistemology 15, 25, 155
Ethical 4, 26, 45, 55, 127
Ethical monitoring 56
Ethics committee 59
Ethnographic. See ethnography
Ethnography 28, 34, 109, 112, 115
Ethno-radiographer 27
European image quality criteria 65
Evening drinks 129
Existential phenomenology 116
Exit strategy 172

Exogenous variable 84
Experimental 84, 89
External validity 98

Fabricate 56
Fairness 163
Field diary 37
Field notes 7, 130
Filtered back projection 101
Final contact 180
FNF 101
Focus groups 9, 12, 48, 53, 133, 148, 151
Foundationalism 16, 29
FPF 101
Frequency distribution 102
Friendliness 177
Friendships 134
Fun 172

Gap analysis 38
Gatekeepers 48, 51, 138, 140
General imaging 7, 17, 83
Generalized linear regression 93
Generalizability 12
Generalization 8, 42, 88, 91, 99, 105, 111
Going native 129
Good behaviour 177
Goodness fit 103
Grounded theory 26, 30, 109, 117

Hawthorne effect 123
Hermeneutic phenomenology 115
Hidden ethnography 136
Histogram 95
Honesty 139, 145
Hostile 6, 52, 58, 135
Hounsfield unit 69
Human observer 79
Human perception 95
Hyper-research 147
Hypocrisy 158
Hypothesis test 93
Hypothetical-deduction 19

IAEA 86
ICRP 94
Ideological norms 112
Illegal 50
Image quality criteria 65
Image reconstruction algorithms 94
Image segmentation 95
Imaging parameters 66
Imaging protocol 73
Immersion 6, 24, 113, 129
Impact 24, 33, 51, 58, 81, 118

Inaccuracy 46, 69
Incognito 53
Independent variable 68, 75
Inductive 24, 35, 50, 98, 112
Infants 128
Inferential statistics 93
Informed consent 46, 53
Interobserver variability 82
Interpretative phenomenological analysis 155
Interpretivism 11, 17, 22, 118, 123
Interval scale 81
Interventional effect 84
Interview schedule 131
Interview transcripts 40, 149, 151
Interviewees 133
Interviews 9, 49, 85, 116, 120, 130, 131
Intrusion 136
Ionizing chamber dosimeter 9
Ionizing radiation 16, 23, 28, 35, 51, 75, 151
Iterative image reconstruction 101
Iterative process 150

Joy 6
Justice 47, 48

Kurt Lewin 119
Kurtosis 95

LDRL 95
Lead protection 111, 150
Leaving the field 4, 54, 56, 136, 171
Legitimacy 16
Level of confidence 70
Liberate 119
Lifeenhancing 119
Likelihood observer 102
Likert scale 65
Linear nonthreshold (LNT) 35
Linear regression 93
Linguistic 117
Link function 103
Literature review 36, 41, 70, 90
Lived experience 110
Locum radiographer 129, 177
Logical positivism 19
Logistic function 69
Low dose regime 71
Low impact 163
LSS 72

Magnetic resonance imaging 17, 114
Maintaining access 51
Maintaining good relationships 171
Majorities voice 162

Bronisław Malinowski 112, 137
Mammography 111, 116
Manuscript 151
Mathematical analysis 63
Mathematical operation 68
Mean drug effect 100
Measurement process 79
Measurement scales 81
Mediators 133
Medical torture 46
Medicine 109, 113, 174
Member checking 56, 157
Memoing 165
Metaanalysis 70
Metaphysical 19
Methodological surprises 162
Milligray 79
Mini-conclusions 41
Moral 45, 50, 56, 128
Motivation 1
Multiconstructive experiences 160
Multi-sited fieldwork 160
Multi-sited research 136, 150

Narrative 2, 15, 25, 40, 45, 132, 147, 152
National Institute of Standard and Technology 87
National Radiation Protection Board 87
Natural law 20, 63
Natural sciences 2, 19, 111
Natural setting 111, 113, 127
Near misses 153
Nonexperimental design 67
Nonparametric statistics 102
Note taking 140, 148
Null hypothesis 39, 59
Nuremberg Code 46
NVivo 147

Objectives 4, 8, 39, 43, 66, 84, 102
Objectivist 16, 29
Observation 3, 17, 22, 35, 68, 72, 85, 111, 113, 114, 128, 130
Observational notes 146
Observational surveys 85
Observer as participant 129
Ontology 15, 20, 137, 155
Open access 87
Open-ended questions 131
Operability 89
Operating theatre 120
Oppress 25
Optical density function 95
Ordinal regression 82
Ordinal scale 82
Originality 2, 6, 26, 36, 42

Otherness 137
Outspokenness 134
Overt 8, 53, 115, 121, 130, 140

PACS 79
Paediatric patients 128
Paradigm shift 3
Paradigm war 3
Parametric statistics 97
Participant as observer 129
Participant information sheet 48
Participant observation 113
Participatory action research 119
Patients capacity 48
Peer reviewed journals 66
Performance test 93
Person centred care 52
Personal diary 37
Personalized dose prescription 69
Pessimism 8
Phantom sizes 81
Phases I and II 73
Phases III and IV 73
PhD 3, 11, 17, 30, 34, 41, 58, 173, 179
Phenomenological analysis 116
Phenomenology 34, 115, 116
Philosophical lens 8, 117
Philosophy of science 15
Philosophy of social science 15
Photographs 50
Photon beam filtration 94
Pictures 3
Pilot studies 79
PIS. See participant information sheet
Placebo 59, 82
Plagiarism 56
Pluralist 18, 29
Policy 58, 111, 123, 164, 175
Positionality 9, 48, 127, 136, 137, 158
Positivism 7, 19, 29, 112
Postmodern ethnography 28
Postmodern shift 178
Postmodernism 10, 26, 30
Postmodernist See postmoderism
Post-positivism 16, 20
Power imbalance 118
Pragmatism 16, 27, 30
Precision 88
Primary data 36, 40
Privacy 46, 59, 120
Probability density distribution 94
Pseudonyms 148
Psychological measurement 94
Psychometric function 95
Psychophysics studies 95

Quantum physics 94
Quasiexperimental studies 68
Questionnaire 79
Quick exit 172

Radiation dose 64, 65, 72, 81
Radiation protection 67, 71, 82
Radical positivism 19
Radiographic appreciation 164
Radiographic imaging 19
Radiography student 35, 137
Radiological diagnosis 9
Radiologist 21, 65
Radiosensitive 30, 35
Radiotherapy 15
Randomised recruitment 75
Randomized controlled trial 75
Rapid ethnography 114
Rapport 114, 128, 173
Ratio scale 79
Raw data 146
Rayleigh scattering 69
Receiver operating characteristic (ROC) 71
Reflexive. See Reflexivity
Reflexive practitioner 176
Reflexivity 136
Regulatory requirements 56
Rehabilitation 17
Reliability 67
Research culture 9
Research design 17
Research Excellence Framework 174
Research opportunity 36
Research problem 39
Research proposal 42
Research questions 43, 47, 73, 90, 110, 120, 132, 172
Researcher bias 162
Retrospective studies 72

Salami publication 57
Self-educative journey 120
Semi-structured interview 131
Sensitive 6, 51, 131, 137, 148, 172
Sensitivity 47
Sequential phase 49
Serum caffeine levels 68
Shorthand representations 130
Sigmoid curve 95
Significance level 97
Size effect 66
Skewness 95
Slopes 96
Social circles 129
Social constructionism 16
Social media 50, 178, 181

Solitary pulmonary nodules 101
Sorting 145
Source to image distance 130
Spiritual 26
SPSS 97
Stagnant 9
Standard deviation 89
Standardised protocol 85
Statistical analysis 7, 70
Statistical inference 3
Statistical power 97
Statistical signal detection theory 102
Statistical test 102
Step function 98
Stochastic response 71
Storing 146
Story 152
Storytelling 153
Structured interviews 131
Subculture 113
Subjectivity 139
Suboptimum radiographic practices 151
Supervisors 4, 34, 35, 51, 118, 177
Supervisory meetings 161
Survey 91, 148, 149, 164, 165, 174, 176, 177, 178, 179, 184
Survey screening 15
Surveys 70
Swimming pool 5
Symbolic interactionism 110, 118
Systematic review 70

T-test 82
Tactical authenticity 164
Technological 10, 114, 147
The alternative hypothesis 100
The Discovery of Grounded Theory 117
Theatre radiography 120
Thematic analysis 151, 153
Theological 19
Theoretical sampling 154
Theoretical saturation 154
Therapeutic tool 134
Thick description 159
Time series 83
Tissue response 94
Toilet 130
Tokenistism 161

Toxic 10
Training data 98
Transcendental 115
Transcript 148
Transcription 134, 141, 146, 157
Transferability 159
Treatment control function 95
Triangulation 159
True experimental studies 68
True-negative fraction 100
True-positive fraction 101
Trust 129, 138
Trustworthiness 145
Tuskegee syphilis experiment 46
Two-group posttests 83
Type I error 100
Type II error 100

Ultrasound 174
Uncertainty 64
Unethical 46, 50, 55, 63, 74
Ungeneralizable 5
United Nations scientific committee for radiation protection, 94
United science 2, 178
Unpredictability 47, 55
Unspoken reticence 135
Unstructured interviews 141

Validity 16, 67, 71, 82, 88, 90, 112
Values 17
Variability 89
Verbal consent 54
Verbal diagnosis 49
Verbatim 112, 123
Video recordings 148
Videos 180
Visual grading scale 65

Webbased questionnaire 86
Weibull function 96
Wilcoxon matched-pair test 102
World Health Organisation 47
World Medical Association 47
Writing up 150

X-ray experiment 3, 34, 66
X-ray room 9, 41, 52, 113, 172

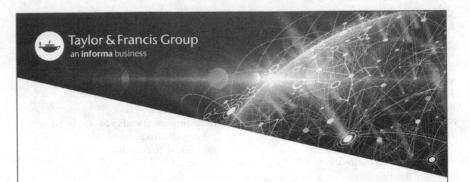

Printed in the United States
by Baker & Taylor Publisher Services